CREATING AN ABUNDANT PRACTICE

A Spiritual and Practical Guide
for Holistic Practitioners
and Healing Centers

By
Andrea Adler

Second edition, revised
Copyright@2003 Andrea Adler
Second printing - 2005

Library of Congress Cataloging-in-Publication Data
Adler, Andrea, 2003
Creating an Abundant Practice:
A Spiritual and Practical Guide
for Holistic Practitioners and Healing Centers
p.   cm.

ISBN # 0-9715243-1-9

andrea@holisticpr.com
www.HolisticPR.com

Formally published under the title:
PR For the Holistic Healer, 2001

Book design by Melanie Pahlmann
Cover design by Gene Krachkel

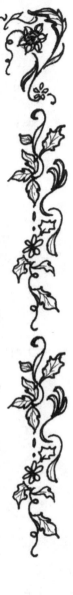

In dedication:

to

Gurumayi Chidvilasananda,

for her endless, loving

encouragement

&

to all the gifted, compassionate

practitioners in the world.

TABLE OF CONTENTS

INTRODUCTION

Dear health practitioners and healing centers,

Congratulations! How courageous of you to pick up this book, hold it in your hands and consider the fact that it may provide you with the knowledge and insight you are seeking. I'm confident that it will answer many of your questions regarding the topic of promoting and marketing your practice. I also hope that you embrace what it has to offer, and that it puts you at ease — and at the same time lights a fire in your solar plexus, so that you may begin to implement the exercises and tools with confidence and enthusiasm.

This book is the second edition to *PR for the Holistic Healer: A Handbook on Promoting and Marketing Your Practice*. The reason I changed the name to *Creating an Abundant Practice* is because, although marketing and PR is what most practitioners need to know, many of you would walk right by the book without ever picking it up and giving it a try. Realizing the words *PR* and *marketing* were a turn -off to you made me crazy. It made my heart sink. However, this little episode showed me how important the title of a book can be. And if it's the wrong title, which it clearly was, we'd better change it. So, I did.

I loved the word *abundance* and wanted to incorporate it into the new title, as I loved the way it sounded; the way it uplifted me when I heard it; the way it expanded my thoughts about money, wealth. I thought about the word for several days and acknowledged that abundance was not only about financial success and how much we can accumulate and spend on ourselves and our loved ones. Abundance is about a "life perspective," a balance of the spiritual and practical aspects of our lives. Combining the words *abundance* and *holistic* represented, at least to me, the sum totality of who we can become as human beings.

This book is dedicated to those holistic practitioners who strive for that kind of abundance. It is dedicated to those who channel and offer their gifts and move with the wind of the spirit and their own inner currents; who give of themselves wholeheartedly to a society that is just now beginning to open up to what you all have to offer. My heart goes out to you, and therefore I have dedicated my life to supporting your efforts.

WHY I SUPPORT YOU

For as long as I can remember and for most of my adult life I have used complementary medicines to cure or rebalance my emotional and physical body. When I was old enough to know the difference between allopathic and holistic approaches, allopathic methods had little appeal for me. Complementary forms of healing became the only way I chose to heal myself. I vividly remember friends' and family members' thinking I was crazy for experimenting and trusting these (as they thought) "voodoo" methods of treatment; they would try their hardest to talk me out of using them on myself and my son. But I knew in my heart these methods would heal me, and time after time, my instincts were proved right.

There were special remedies placed under my tongue to restore my anxious mind, flower essences for my troubled soul, finger pressure applied to meridians to treat a problematic colon. When I returned home from a trip to India, I found myself eating and eating, gaining weight and not feeling nourished. An iridologist took one look in my eyes and said, "You're eating for five hundred — parasites, that is; no wonder you're not feeling nourished." After a few acupuncture treatments and a month's supply of homeopathic remedies, those little critters were gone.

I could go on and on detailing all the unconventional and yet remarkable ways I have been healed, be it through crystals, needles, tinctures, your hands. But if I were to indulge in the praise you deserve, this book would become a 600-page testimonial about how much I've appreciated your contributions to my good health. It would become a thank-you to your healing hands, your kind hearts and great wisdom. And although these are the reasons I sat down to write this new edition in the first place, the fact is, the book has another purpose.

Creating an Abundant Practice is a step-by-step guide on how to create wholeness where there is separation; how to envision the future of your dreams; how to ensure the longevity of your healing center; how to garner partnerships and cultivate all kinds of exciting exposure — and how to approach these initiatives as a spiritual practice and as healing in themselves. This book will provide you with sample resumés, bios, press releases and questionnaires to study and use as examples, so there's little room for doubt. Firsthand anecdotes and practical advice will help you navigate unexpected or difficult situations; self-evaluation tools will aid you in pinpointing and realizing your career and lifestyle goals.

I have tried to create an easy-to-read reference that will help you to gain the strength and courage necessary to thrive as both a healer and a business owner, as a healing center and a commercial entity and, in so doing, help you to integrate these two aspects of your practice into your daily activities.

In hindsight, my first book, *PR for the Holistic Healer,* was a labor of love. This new edition became a fascinating exercise in letting go, becoming the channel for new information to flow, gracefully — from my heart onto the page. It was my intention not only to share with you the practical ways in which to bring abundance into your practice, but to convey philosophical ideas that will provide you with a strong, vivid subtext to support your journey. Personally, I can't create anything of value in my life without a spiritual subtext. When I try to do so, everything seems dry, hollow, without essence.

Therefore, as you will see, the first part of the book conveys these philosophical approaches. The second half of the book is of a more practical, how-to nature.

As you travel through these pages there will inevitably be challenges that will come up for you. Please, go through them regardless of your resistance.

"Fearlessness," Mahatma Gandhi said, "is the first prerequisite of a spiritual life."

Fear is a healthy motivator. It can be the catalyst for moving us beyond our wildest dreams. When unacknowledged, however, fear transforms itself into depression. This, I have come to understand, is the soul manifesting itself, crying out that it wants to change, begging us for our permission.

It behooves us all to face our fear — look it straight in the face, talk to it, have compassion for it, embrace it, then tell it we understand why it's there; only then can we begin to watch it dissolve, as we begin to take action.

Trusting that the actions we take will prove to be successful will bring about fearlessness.

The tools are here, ready for you to use. It's up to you to try them, to imbibe them, master them. Once that's accomplished, I guarantee your practice and your life will inevitably shine with heavenly blessings.

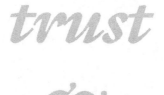

trust

&

fearlessness

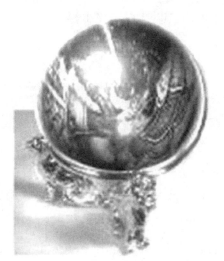

CHAPTER 1

ENVISIONING YOUR FUTURE

Envisioning Your Future

If you don't have a clear vision of where you want to be,
you probably aren't going to get there.
~ Ti Caine

An extraordinary meeting took place a short time ago that changed the way I looked at every aspect of my life: my family, my friends, my intimate relationships, and my work. The meeting was with my future.

This meeting was not an accident. It never is. It's just that I'd never placed much importance on it. Oh, I knew it was there, but it was "in the future," so I thought I had plenty of time to think about it.

What I have come to *realize* is how much our contemplation of the future brings about the present. And depending on the quality and clarity of that vision, it can literally become a magnet that pulls us right smack into its magnificent vortex.

What I have come to *experience* is that when we connect with this deep internal flame of genuine passion and undeniable inspiration, when we reside in the place of knowing that our future is real, standing right before us, and that all we have to do is believe in it, walk into it, and it will be ours — we can live fully, joyously in the magnificent present.

I must admit, I did not jump into this FutureVisioning™ concept with all fours when first introduced to it. On the contrary, I had a lot of resistance. I actually kicked and screamed during several telephone conversations with Ti Caine, the metaphysician who had turned me on to this concept, before deciding to go through with this process I'd heard so much about.

These thoughts came up very strongly:
Doesn't the future spring naturally from the present?
Isn't it all karma anyway?

I mean, I'd spent thousands of hours meditating so I could learn to live in and appreciate the moment. I'd spent years chanting, to open my heart so I'd stop lamenting the past. I was an avid reader of *Awakening,* a Buddhist magazine, Ram Dass's classic *Be Here Now,* and *The Power of Now* and *Practicing the Power of Now,* by Eckhardt Tolle. Thirty years had been spent trying to incorporate these teachings into my thoughts and actions. So attached was I to living in the moment that the mere thought of thinking about the future seemed — well, frivolous. Setting this huge part of me aside to focus on something that seemed, for the most part, to be out of my control was a bit much for this highly sensitive, disciplined *yogini.*

And yet, I had to look at my life. I was a single parent. My son had just left for college, I'd moved out of our beautiful home in Westchester, New York to recoup expenses. The apartment I was now living in was dark and depressing and the neighborhood was not one I particularly enjoyed. And even though I was meditating and chanting and focusing on the moment, even though I was in excellent health and my first book had come out with good reviews, even though I had wonderful, loving friends — my life sucked.

There was this knot in my gut, knowing I could do more, be more, but I didn't know how to claim it. There seemed to be no light at the end of the dark hallway I was sitting in — only fog.

After my first FutureVisioning™ session, I experienced an incredible new awareness of myself. I was able to see my future with amazing clarity, in shining, luminous, living color. It was everything I'd wanted it to be. I was married to a loving, beautiful man and living in a spacious home. The climate where my new home was situated was warm and dry with lots of sunshine — clearly not New York. My son was coming to visit us on holidays. My work was thriving. I had interesting, creative friends. I was writing books and presenting workshops all over the world. I was so happy.

Now, I don't want to mislead you. I had had glimpses of this dream before this session; only now it seemed very real, very concrete, and very attainable.

What had become clear to me now was that if I didn't start building a relationship with my future, the present was not going to change — at least, not in the ways that would bring about the results my soul longed for. And the trick was, not to live in the future constantly or I'd miss the sweet moments of the present. I began to understand that all the meditation and chanting practices I had been doing were fine. Actually, quite helpful. They didn't have to be put aside. The years had certainly not been wasted. There was just something else I had to do: I had to balance these practices along with maintaining the vision of my future.

So I started to really focus on what I wanted my future to look like. I began to see it and feel it in the greatest of detail. And within only a few days, I began to feel lighter and lighter, freer from the current constructs I'd created in my mind. I began to experience why I was blocked. And then, like the infinity symbol, with the loop going out into the future first and then coming back and out into the future again, the FutureVisioning™ exercise showed me that by experiencing my future first, returning to my inner child to heal some core issues that were blocking my path, and going out into the future again, I could live in the moment in a whole new way.

Because my attention was now on this luminous future that I'd seen and felt as if I could touch, I no longer experienced the present as being so miserable. The present began to transform itself in a way that I actually felt the molecules in my body change; the quicksand that had been drowning me for months let go its hold. The fog lifted and my old companion, joy, had returned.

I began to move quickly into my vision, effortlessly, gracefully. It was only a few weeks later that I'd made the decision to go on a two-month journey through the Southwest to find a new home. It was clear to me that I'd needed a change from New York. I began my sojourn by visiting a friend in Santa Barbara, and then went to visit another friend in Tucson. As beautiful as Tucson was, as much as I loved the climate and the people, it didn't resonate fully with me. It didn't feel like home.

So I visited Prescott, Sedona, Phoenix, Albuquerque. None of these cities felt right for me to live in. It wasn't until I arrived in Santa Fe that I knew: this was the place I wanted to settle into. This was where I was going to plant new roots. Everything came together for me there, like magic: a house, workshops, people I had common interests with. It was truly amazing! I felt like I had stepped into the reality of my own vision.

WHY FEAR CAN BE A MOTIVATOR

When I returned to New York, the entire trip seemed like a dream. I began to doubt that I could actually go through with this move. Fear, anxiety, worry popped up like old enemies wanting to take over my psyche. I found I had to think more deeply about this whole FutureVisioning™ experience. Athletes, I recalled, had been using visualization to win matches for years. Yogis had visualized their bodies as stoves to fend off brutal winters for lifetimes. With all my years of meditating and visualizing my body as a divine temple, if I couldn't envision and experience an awesome future for myself, who was I to teach anyone anything? My very fear gave me the impetus to look beyond it.

HOLDING THE VISION

In Robert Moss's book *Dreaming True,* he makes reference to ancient Polynesian navigators who managed to sail thousands of miles across the Pacific without a compass or instruments of any kind. Instead, they brought an old-time navigator, a Waymaker, on board, to train their crew. The Waymaker taught the crew how to listen to the waves, talk to the winds and follow the stars. When they were facing the general direction of their destination, he told them to close their eyes and use all their senses, to taste it, to smell it, touch it. When the vision was alive for them, he instructed them: "Hold the vision in your mind, or else you will be lost."

It was clear by the description in the story that had the ancient Polynesians spent their time worrying about the high winds or the stormy seas, they never would have reached their destination. They did reach their destination of Hawaii, and only because they had held the vision.

Reading about Waymaking proved to me once again that we can dream our dream into manifestation — into the physical world. By holding our vision, we can create a magnetism that draws our destination to us.

Not until I put this practice into my own life did I begin to understand the significance of this process. When I realized that every single thought we have can take us either closer to our future or further away, this became an amazing epiphany. After the move to the Southwest, seeing adventure coming back into my life, and the return of the magic that I'd experienced as a child, feeling my work accelerated and my passion for living heightened, I knew this was something I had to offer my readers. Because the truth is, there is no end to the benefits from this process. It's for anyone who has a future!

And, since we're all in the same business of helping people create better futures, I urge you to experiment with the FutureVisioning™ exercise. Explore the possibilities for yourself, first. Then, if you wish, and when it is appropriate, try it with your own clients. Can you imagine? If they see a healthy future for themselves, your job will be so much easier.

THE FUTUREVISIONING™ EXERCISE

Take a comfortable posture, with writing materials close to hand.

Close your eyes. Take a deep breath; fill your lungs with all the wonderful air that surrounds you.

Let it out slowly.

Take another deep breath. As you breathe in, ask for clarity and wisdom from your heart.

Allow your breath to exhale slowly.

As you breathe out, ask yourself: If I were to design my ideal future, what would it look like? If gave myself total permission to dream the most magnificent future I could dream, what would the image feel like, look like?

You are the master of your fate. Allow your imagination to soar beyond the room, beyond time, beyond space. And know that you have a choice: to walk through one of five different doors. You can walk through the "awful door," the "mediocre door," the "good door," the "better door,"or the "awesome door."

Once you have selected the door you want to step through, see what your most incredible future could be like if you allowed it to manifest right now.

Take your time. Really see this future, breathe into it with your mind and heart. Breathe into it with your body. Feel it, taste it. Experience it in as much detail as possible. Hold nothing back. See the whole picture. Your entire life. Not just your practice. See your intimate relationships, your family, your friends, your pets.

Breathe in deeply; let the air out slowly.

When you have this vision of your most amazing future, open your eyes and write it down if you like. Then continue the exercise with your eyes closed.

Breathe in again. Only this time, imagine yourself one year from now: Once again, select one of the doors to walk through: the awful door, the mediocre door, the good door, the better door, or the awesome door. Select any one of the five doors and walk through, and see what your life could be like one year from now.

See it in as much detail as possible. See what changes have been made from the year you are now in. What has stayed the same?

Is your residence the same?

Are you still married? Single? In love?

Most importantly, feel the quality of the year.

Breathe in deeply again; let it out slowly. Take another deep breath.

Now, as you breathe out, imagine yourself three years from now. Select and walk through one of the five doors. And imagine what your life could be like three years from today. Ask yourself: What changes have been made? Am I living in the same place? Am I practicing in the same location? Am I traveling, lecturing? See your life in as much detail as possible and see the year, smell it, taste it. Let your heart guide you toward your deepest yearnings.

Breathe in deeply again; let it out slowly.

Take another deep breath.

As you breathe out, imagine yourself five years from now. Select one of the five doors to walk through and visualize what your life could be like in five years' time. Step into the picture and look at the changes, if any, and the places where things have stayed the same. See the whole picture, listen for sounds, look for colors. Take everything in and experience the satisfaction of your heart's desire.

Breathe in deeply again; let it out slowly.

Take another deep breath.

Now, envision your life as an elderly man or woman. Where are you living? What are you doing? Are you enjoying life in your elder years? Are you alone, or are you surrounded by family and friends?

Experience the inner feelings as well as the outer circumstances. See the details, feel the details.

When you have all four visions in your mind, open your eyes and write them down. If one or more of the moments in time was not clear for you, do not be concerned. It may not be the time for you to have a vision or any visual experience. Trust that too.

WE CHOOSE OUR DESTINY

What I love about this exercise is that if there is any part of the future we are unhappy about, we can change it. If we see ourselves as an old lady or an old man who is not in the best of health, we can change our vision. We can see that old lady, that old man, as vibrant and happy. If we don't want to go through numerous relationships before finding the right one, we can find the right one right away. If we're open to it. It's all a matter of choice. Our choice. It's our life.

Whatever vision it is we create, we need to hold it in our heart, meditate on it, see it with great clarity. For the closer we hold it, the easier it will be for us to manifest. Regardless of the distractions and unexpected turbulence of events that come along, regardless of detours and delays, we need to hold the vision in our mind's eye, and be ready to sail on its currents.

When we are excited about where we are going, we inevitably provide better service; we're more motivated to do what it takes; we are open metaphysically and spiritually to the magic we are moving toward and the magic of the process itself. This new paradigm for success, this turning point in human psychology, will not only bring you the abundance you desire for your practice; it will bring to you an abundant life.

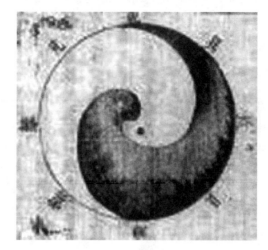

CHAPTER 2

CREATING WHOLENESS

Creating Wholeness

Like the proverbial pebble dropped into a still pond,
the shifts of consciousness we make in our personal lives send out tiny but
important waves that ripple over the surface of the whole.

~ Shakti Gawain

There seems to be a distinctive thought process that occurs among healing practitioners whenever I broach the subject of "getting the word out there" about their practice. What is interesting is that the same kind of thinking occurs when I discuss this very topic with musicians, actors and artists. Their thoughts go something like this: "I'm a practitioner, not a businessperson," "I'm a musician, not a promoter," I'm an actor, I can't market myself."

It's as if these practitioners and artists believe that the ability to aid in the healing process, or the desire to perform, cannot coexist within the same person with the art of promotion. It's as if people in these professions believe they lack wholeness — that there is a separation between their artistic or healing endeavor and their ability to promote and market their profession.

When this feeling of separation comes up for any of us, it keeps us from experiencing the magnificent truth of who we are and what we are capable of achieving.

As long as we experience this disconnect, this split in our psyches, we will be removed from alignment, from our soul's calling, and from entering the future of our dreams. When we can come to the place of knowing that this disconnect is not a permanent condition, that there is a creative, noninvasive cure, we can open ourselves to the possibility of change and trust that this change will stay with us, as long as we remain committed to the journey. It all begins with the willingness to learn, the desire to practice and integrate new information.

WE LEARN THROUGH REPETITION

Just as healing takes place on all levels within the body, mind, and spirit simultaneously, the same is true for learning. If we are not open to receiving on all levels, we block the process of absorption.

One of the best ways to learn anything is by repeating the desired information over and over. It is the repetition that ultimately makes the new data familiar. Whether we're learning to tie our shoes, developing a new swim stroke or adapting to a new computer (something I'm having to do at this very moment), the trick is to be patient with ourselves, to allow the new information to seep into our brains, into our bodies and into our feeling, until it becomes so familiar it becomes second nature.

"The brain actually makes new connections during the learning process," says Sherri Senné, a consultant for innovative learning strategies. "Neurons that fire together, wire together, and they create new learning patterns. That is why repetition is so valuable — in fact, crucial. We are continually remaking ourselves anew: body, mind, brain, and spirit. But even with that understanding, there is still much more going on during the process of learning — but it's happening throughout the body, at different receptors sites on all kinds of cells, not just at the brain's synapses or through the cells of the central nervous system."

WE LEARN BY INTEGRATING

The more often we repeat the new information, the easier it becomes to integrate it into our daily regime. The more a person practices massage with sensitivity to the energy and motional nuances of the body/mind they are treating, the better a massage therapist they become. The more knowledge a practitioner amasses about the subtleties of essential oils, the better their service to their client. It's the same protocol for learning the tools of PR and marketing: repetition and integration. By repeating and integrating, you create a synthesis for learning.

THE FIRST STEP

Once we take the first step, no matter how difficult the new information may seem to be, and open ourselves to new stimuli, the next step becomes easier and the next step even easier!

Taoist philosopher Lao-tzu (604 -531 BCE) said,
"A journey of a thousand miles must begin with a single step."

A friend of mine was, and still is, an outstanding speaker. He can speak eloquently for hours about the most amazing, complex psychological and physiological topics. However, when it comes time to writing down his thoughts on paper, he is completely lost. He doesn't know where to begin. Apparently he'd experienced this writing block since childhood. When I explained to him that the act of writing is a skill, a muscle that needs to be developed through exercise, he said, "Wow, I've never heard it described that way before. I never saw writing as a skill. I've only seen it as a laborious chore." I asked him to do some simple mind-body exercises to help integrate the learning process for one hour every day. No more, no less.

One of the exercises I suggested was to sit in the lotus posture and meditate for at least twenty minutes in the morning — before he starts his daily activities. This practice would help him slow down his thoughts and provide him with the clarity he needs. After meditation, I asked him to write for at least half an hour. He told me he would give it a try and get back to me.

A few weeks later he called me and told me he was floored. He was actually writing and enjoying it for the first time in his life. He said he'd set up a daily discipline for himself, was doing the exercises repeatedly, and writing for a half hour every morning. "It wasn't easy in the beginning," he said; "it brought up all kinds of stuff from my youth. But I kept doing it and the half hour turned into one hour and then into two. Today, I wrote the beginning of a short piece that could eventually become an article. This is very cool."

My friend was able to move out of an old mindset that had kept him contracted for years. After seeing the act of writing from a different perspective (nonpersonal), after courageously taking the first step, he was able to let down his guard, become the receiver — as this is a receptive process, not a doership one — and adopt the new skill.

When we understand that the art of
promoting and marketing is the same creative energy
that stimulates us to write, to create mastery on stage,
to become a channel for healing, we can drop our resistance
and draw upon this force to lead us into the
flow of mastering our profession.

THE CHALLENGE FOR NEW PRACTITIONERS

I've known several people, as I'm sure you do, who have transitioned from being real-estate agents or lawyers, secretaries or accountants, to becoming holistic practitioners: acupuncturists, hypnotherapists or massage therapists.

For those practitioners who have consciously worked on themselves to evolve spiritually, the transition from their past profession to their new one can be seamless. For others it can be devastatingly difficult. For instance, those people who have not done the necessary inner work may experience a certain degree of discomfort, even culture shock. Neophyte practitioners who may have been accustomed to a corporate structure must now adapt to an entirely new mindset, a new way of being. Their previous way of communicating no longer works and this shift can cause quite a bit of anxiety. The hard-shell surface and automatic behavioral response that might have worked in the day-to-day grind of the corporate world no longer serves in the classroom or the treatment room where healing takes place. This new work requires using heart, body, and mind in chorus. Time and again, practitioners need to reach inside themselves and use their sensitivity, their intuition, and their feeling.

BESIDES THE EMOTIONAL SHIFT, THERE IS THE INTELLECTUAL SHIFT

One woman I know who had been a housewife and mother to three children for thirteen years had so much anxiety while taking her midterms for massage school that she had to drop out of her classes before the end of the first semester. She simply could not learn all that was required of her. She felt awful after spending so much time in school and so much money on tuition. She just wasn't used to using this part of her brain and it became more of a strain to her than a pleasurable new vocation.

In addition to learning all that is required in school, practitioners must continue to learn new modalities to increase their marketability as well as their effectiveness. They also have to educate themselves on how to promote and market themselves. This is quite a bundle of information to digest.

OUR BRAIN CAN LEARN NEW INFORMATION MORE EASILY BY EXERCISING ITSELF IN NEW WAYS

So how can we make it easier on ourselves to learn new information and integrate it into our lives so our practices flourish? First off, we can remain flexible and pliable. The minute we become contracted, we stop the flow of receiving everything, including the ability to learn. We can practice repetition and integration. We can also do exercises that stimulate our brains — to keep them in shape. In the same way that we exercise our bodies to be strong in order to have more energy, we

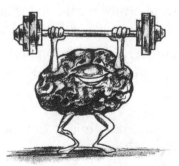

can exercise our brains so they become receptive to new stimuli.

BRAIN GYMNASTIC DRILLS

As a way to move out of former ways of thinking and to prepare the imagination for new possibilities, to help integrate and revitalize our overall condition, Melvin D. Saunders, author of *100% Brain Usage to Higher Consciousness,* suggests we begin the process of stimulating our brains. One way to accomplish this is by practicing any one or all of the following seven "brain gymnastic" drills. (Not to be confused with the Dennisons' Brain Gyms®, a series of muscle-activation techniques for brain integration.) The beauty of these exercises is such that each drill touches upon a different area of our brain. Brain gymnastic drills are also a lot of fun:

1. Get used to your body in new ways. Switch your handedness and comb your hair, brush your teeth, stir your coffee or do other simple tasks with your nondominant hand; or close your eyes and sense your way slowly around a room. Get truly conscious of the sounds and smells in the space around you. Or use your feet to pick up things, flush the toilet or close a door. Read a page in a book holding it horizontally and then upside down!

2. Where you would usually criticize someone, find something to compliment him or her on instead! Suspend your judgment about that person and view him or her as simply another human being with different viewpoints from your own.

3. Look in your refrigerator briefly, but thoroughly. Then close the door and enumerate the items contained therein. Do the same with a room of your house, a storefront window, or a

detailed picture on the wall.

4. For five minutes every day, put yourself in another person's shoes and view things from their perspective; see how life is for them compared to how it is for you.

5. Whenever you catch yourself worrying, doubting, or looking down on yourself, think instead of the future you want for yourself — in complete detail — and affirm to yourself the achievement of the same. Replay this positive inner movie whenever negative thoughts intrude during your day.

6. At the end of every daily hour, review what's happened to you during the previous 60 minutes. This is good practice for getting more mindful throughout your day. At day's end, mentally review all the events that have happened to you through-out the day up to your present point. Memory gaps about your day's events reveal unconscious moments.

7. To develop flexibility and adaptability to change in your life, do something different every day. Shop at a different store. Take a different route home. Bake a pie or a loaf of bread. Involve yourself in a new game or sport, like roller-skating, bowling, karate or skydiving. Introduce yourself to a new neighbor. Sameness every day is a death knell to your brain. For bringing more of your brain into play, diverse stimulation is the key. It also gets you unstuck from habits and ruts that are bringing you unfavorable results.

TURN THE EXERCISES INTO A WAY OF LIFE

Please, do not just read through these seven steps and fool yourself into thinking that you've accomplished them. Really try them. These exercises have helped many people more than once to move out of old patterns of thinking. These drills have stimulated imaginations and provided opportunities for expansion and discovery that others like yourself would not have been able to explore had they not tried them.

Adopt one or two into your day-to-day schedule and see what happens. I'm sure it'll be fascinating to watch the subtle shift that takes place. You'll see, all of a sudden you'll try new things, meet new people, explore new situations you never thought you'd experience. The same holds true for healing centers. Especially when everyone in the center decides to consciously create change. There will be more cohesiveness, a heightened awareness of others, and a more harmonious environment.

When the spiritual, emotional, and practical applications of these understandings become integrated, all of our resistances dissolve. When we give ourselves permission to let go of old behaviors that no longer serve us, we are able to play and have fun with new forms of self-expression. The experience of ultimate freedom will be ours. We'll be able to stand back and watch how simply, how elegantly our efforts will bear the fruits we desire.

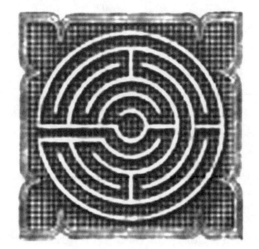

CHAPTER 3

DEFINING HEALING CENTERS

Defining Healing Centers

*There are two aspects of individual harmony: the harmony between
body and soul, and the harmony between individuals.*

~ Hazrat Inayat Khan

As much as we try to achieve the goal of "Know thyself" through
various spiritual practices, the capacity to build trust and power in
working with others is the result of building intimate relationships.
My work with practitioners and healing centers, combined with my
twenty-six-year practice of meditation, has fueled this exploration of
intimacy. At the same time, it is clear to me that while the practice
of meditation brings clarity and connectedness to my core, expan-
siveness to my heart, joy to my soul, it doesn't guarantee healthy
personal relationships.

It's even possible to use meditation, at least during certain peri-
ods in our life, as a way of avoiding intimacy.

ESTABLISH A RELATIONSHIP NARRATIVE

Richard Strozzi Heckler, author of *Holding the Center* — one of the
most magnificent books I've read on relationships — says that to
even start the conversation of commitment in a marriage, for instance,
a couple needs to develop the same story about the reason for the

relationship. In the "relationship narrative" (which is, in fact, the story of the relationship and why two people have come together), each person shares a commitment regarding their common future. They make decisions about what they want their future to look like. This can include having children, buying a house, building a business, living in the country, or choosing a community. The narrative is the relationship center. A major breakdown for most marriages, Strozzi Heckler goes on to say, is that there is not a shared story about what the partners care about. Each has an individual narrative about his or her own life, but not a relationship narrative. Without a relationship narrative, harmony will not reside in the marriage. Differences and conflict will invariably surface and, with no foundation to work from, the marriage will fall apart.

The same is true for healing centers. Unless the people involved are willing to become intimate players in creating an abundant center, committed to making contributions toward the same vision, the road ahead can be filled with differences and conflict. Conflict will arise not only among the people who have founded and are developing the center, it will arise with everyone working within the facility, and even with clients as well.

Energetically, these two qualities can be profoundly subtle and therefore overlooked. Harmony is detected immediately, subliminally, because there is a natural flow of ease and comfort. Discord seeps into the atmosphere insidiously and can remain undetected for years. Unless there is a conscious, ongoing effort among all partners to become clear and honest with each other, the center will never succeed.

CREATING FUSION

A few months ago, I was invited to meet with a healing center in

Chestnut Ridge, New York. I knew the people at the center very well and was quite fond of them, as they were caring, talented practitioners. They had a wonderful reputation for the quality of work performed by each practitioner, but as a center, they lacked proficiency in several areas. Not generating anywhere near the number of clients they knew they could draw, they called me in for a consultation.

I met with three people from the center: one of the founders, a new partner who had recently joined the team, and a part-time secretary who was donating her time in exchange for participating in courses offered there.

We sat in a small circle and talked about their roles, what they had done in the past to market their center, outreach techniques that had worked and hadn't worked; what kinds of people and industries existed within a five- to ten-mile radius that they could draw from. I explained to them the advantages of having a relationship narrative and had each of the participants share what they thought the narration was for them. They spoke about their desire for a quality center: a center that provided a myriad of holistic, alternative applications; a place where people could receive professional care and training. In this case, the participants were on the same page with the "story" of the center.

Next, I invited them to partake in the FutureVisioning™ exercise. After taking them on the one-, three-, and five-year journeys described in Chapter 1, I asked them to open their eyes and describe their vision to the group in detail.

What follows is a summary of their individual visions.

The founder, Paul, a hypnotherapist, saw himself taking on a bigger role as a speaker and workshop presenter in the years ahead, spending less and less time at the center. He also stated that he'd envisioned the center in a new place where there was more pedestrian traffic; the center was currently in an office building off the beaten track and difficult for people to find. Paul also said he saw the new center functioning in an organized fashion, and thriving.

The new partner, Jacques, an energy healer, also saw his role expanding. He saw himself doing more traveling, but still presenting workshops at the center. He said he too saw the center in a new location, although he was more specific. "I saw the center in a large house, across the street from a busy mall. There were lots of people coming through the doors."

The part-time secretary, Norma, somewhat shy because of her tentative role, spoke honestly and said, "I didn't see myself working here in the future. I was coming to the center to take workshops, but that was all." She went on to say, "I saw that we had moved into a Victorian house with a blue door, across the street from a mall, I wasn't sure which mall. And we were very busy."

Everyone sat there with their mouths agape — amazed that they had all seen the same image of their new center in "a house" and how vital and energetic it was. Everybody's guard was down, and intimacy was a welcomed guest. As the awe of the moment settled, it was now my responsibility as the observer of their future to create a strategy by which they could manifest their vision.

I had them close their eyes once again, and asked them to feel what it was like to be in this exciting new space, buzzing with clients coming in and out of sessions and workshops. As they immersed themselves in their new abundance, I asked them what was preventing them from experiencing this abundance right now.

Paul recognized immediately that the center was lacking a nucleus — a single person who could organize the activities of the office, set up appointments, create a marketing and public-relations plan that would be consistent and ongoing.

Jacques admitted that many phone messages had not been answered in a timely way due to lack of personnel. "Continuity is the missing link," he said, "and clients are getting frustrated." He admitted he was too busy to help in these matters. They all nodded in agreement.

Norma, the secretary, said she knew it was time for her to leave her position, as she wanted to return to school. She also knew they needed to hire a full-time employee as she wanted to pursue more educational situations. As an immediate practical concern, she mentioned the need to move the desk, which was sitting in the front of the small lobby and preventing people from walking freely around the room. "It's impossible to talk on the phone when people are in the lobby because of the noise." She suggested moving the desk more toward the back of the room.

CLARITY IS THE GOAL

By having these key people focus on their future, they were able to define current obstacles, clear the way for the future to unfold, and set the stage to prevent the same mistakes from occurring in the new location. This exercise proved to be quite an eye-opener, and as a consequence, everyone was in agreement to take the following steps:

1. They would move the desk toward the back of the room.

2. Paul was to call someone he knew who might be interested in a managerial position, and who might be also be able to

help with marketing and public relations.

3.   Jacques was to call the realtor to start looking for a house in a commercial district.

4.   Paul and Jacques were going to spend spare time driving around looking for possible sites for the new center.

5.   Norma was going to help in the transition and focus more on her education.

In this case, the people involved all had the same relationship narrative, which made the FutureVisioning™ exercise nonthreatening and enjoyable. Because they were willing to examine themselves and be honest about their obstacles as well as their dreams, they were able to make the necessary changes swiftly and move into their vision with ease.

This is not always the case. There are many healing centers and professional organizations that exist in a vacuum and that are for the most part in constant chaos. The fact that a center is "holistic" in intent doesn't mean it can't be dysfunctional. In such a situation, I recommend creating a *mission statement*. The mission statement can act as a vehicle to help bring the relationship narrative to the forefront and provide the center with vision and purpose.

THE NEED FOR VISION AND PURPOSE

No one wants to work for an organization that doesn't have a vision or a purpose. Purpose brings peace and clarity to the workplace. It provides everyone with a reason for being and doing. It sets up parameters for participants to abide by, which ultimately creates a sense of freedom for each person involved, as well as for the group as a whole.

In an effort to demonstrate how a thriving organization can use spiritual and practical guidelines within their manifesto, I've excerpted a mission statement from Lenedra Carroll's' book, *The Architecture of All Abundance.*

While describing her company, *Mani* (the name comes from a Sanskrit term meaning "the wish-fulfilling jewel"), an international initiative that develops, manages, and funds a variety of business ventures, Lenedra points out that there are values that she believes facilitate their projects and interactions. In the mission statement she included words such as *spiritual* and *divine* to provide guidelines but not to create or enforce a particular "spiritual" environment.

In addition to her Mission and Covenant (page 35), Lenedra co-created the Mani Beliefs (page 36).

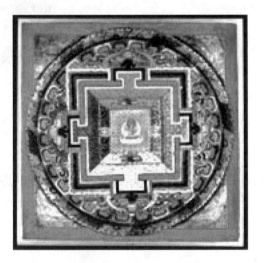

In Tibetan Buddhism, the mandala represents the spiritual embodiment of the Buddha. As for the center, that is the essence. As for the circumference, that is grasping the essence.

MANI MISSION AND COVENANT

It is our Mission to be a powerful global force for positive financial, social, political, and spiritual change. It is our vision and experience that the greatest business success occurs when humanitarian, spiritual, and environmental principals are practiced along with sound business operation. It is our aim to demonstrate this model in the world. We intend to understand what it means to be human beings, in the highest sense, and to integrate this understanding into our being. It is our covenant to:

Serve humanity:
We dedicate our resources and endeavors to be of service. We believe that the blessings of our lives are for the benefit of humanity.

Embody spiritual principles:
We agree to incorporate spiritual virtues such as integrity, peace, humility, love, generosity, compassion, authenticity, and faith into all our actions.

Embrace diversity and support diversity:
We honor diverse beliefs and cultures, each part being vital to the integrity of the whole.

Practice sacred stewardship:
We agree to carefully assess the true costs and contributions of our endeavors and establish balanced exchanges. We are accountable to the whole.

Promote generative prosperity:
Our prosperity is an expression of Divine abundance. We receive it in align-ment with natural laws. We revel in it and share it with joy.

MANI BELIEFS

Self-responsibility

We believe that the organization's aims of global influence, humanitarian service, integrity, and profitability are served when individuals are self-accountable and self-generative, bringing their excellence to the support of the organization.

Expanded Human Potential

We believe it is the responsibility of each team member to transform the workplace by moving beyond limiting behaviors to pioneer processes and actions that expand the individual's capabilities and the organization's accomplishments.

Generous Prosperity

We believe it is possible to be financially prosperous while practicing spiritual principles and serving humanitarian goals. We believe that prosperity must be grounded in stewardship and balanced exchange.

Balanced Implementation

We believe all life requires a rhythm of rest and action. We believe that quiet contemplation, meditation, and prayer are important tools to access stillness and the deep well of creativity to help accomplish our goals.

Relationship with the Divine

We believe an intimate relationship with the Divine is central to joyous and sustainable creativity and responsible productivity.

Be the Difference

We believe it is the challenge and opportunity of our times to translate our values, beliefs, hopes, and ideals into concrete actions.

HEAL THY CENTER ~ FIRST

Take the time to sit down with your core members and look deeply inside your souls and ask yourselves: What do we really want? Individually? Collectively?

When practitioners come together for the sake of partnering, there emerges an extraordinary opportunity for growth and intimacy. This stance of intimacy generate trust, expansion, and creativity.

Each person must, of course, continue with his or her own *sadhana* the personal path of spiritual development. However, when the relationship narrative is consciously expressed and embodied by each member, miraculous healings begin to take place.

When these intimate exchanges of hearts and minds come together, their resonance expands and spreads out into the universe. The energy spreads throughout the physical space, beyond the walls and ceilings, out into the neighborhood, reaching those people who, whether consciously or not, will resonate with your heartfelt message. People will call, walk in the door, set up appointments and demand your attention because you have collectively searched for the truth. There is trust. Everyone in the group has committed themselves to the relationship narrative.

Because your intention is for the highest good, you will never have to be concerned about finding people to treat or to educate; they will be drawn into your center naturally, organically. And not always in the way you expect or imagine.

[The Mani Mission and Mani Beliefs are excerpted from *The Architecture of All Abundance* by Lenedra J.Carroll, ©2001. Reprinted with permission of New World Library, Novato, CA www.newworldlibrary.com]

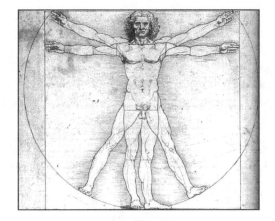

CHAPTER 4

DISTINGUISHING
YOUR PRACTICE

Distinguishing Your Practice

See the world as your self. Have faith in the way things are.
Love the world as your self; then you can care for all things.

~ *Tao te Ching*

While writing the first edition of this book, I had begun to hear stories about how disappointed people were with their therapists' physical space, as well as with their psychic space — how unhappy people were with the treatment and therapeutic experience they were receiving, in general. I heard confessions from clients who felt they'd been mistreated by unconscious or insensitive practitioners.

When I began to interview people about how they felt about their practitioners' spaces, very few people told me they felt totally comfortable and at ease. Only a few were pleased.

I thought this was very strange. It seemed like such a contradiction. How can healing occur in a space that sets up subliminal (or not so subliminal) discomfort? Why would people pay to be put at ease, only to be fighting feelings of unease during the precious time in their therapists' office? Oddly enough, it seemed that when people had a good treatment session and felt comfortable in the space, they tended to keep it to themselves. Which is interesting from a PR standpoint, as it proves once again that negative press spreads more quickly than positive press. What a shame, but it's true!

After spending hours talking to people about their practitioners' spaces — whether chiropractors, massage therapists, or hypnotherapists — I found that I too had some very strong reactions concerning this topic. So, I thought I'd address the issue up front and offer it to your consideration in these pages.

Take a few minutes and contemplate this question before you read on:

*What do my clients experience
when they enter and leave my office?*

YOUR PHYSICAL SPACE

A client walks into your office. What do they feel when they walk through your door? What do they see? What do they smell? What are they listening to? Is the lighting soft and easy on the eyes? Are there candles burning? Is melodic music playing in the background? Not everyone has the same taste in music that you do. What you think is melodic or soothing could drive someone else up the wall. Personally, I never want to hear music that has words when I'm getting a massage. Because I love words so much, I'd spend the entire session concentrating on them and not letting go of my thoughts, which is one of the reasons I've set up the appointment in the first place. I want to let go completely of the mental realm when I'm having a massage or any kind of body treatment. This isn't true for everyone, but it is for many.

Now, some people will not say a word to you about your choice of music at any time during the session, even if they're annoyed by it. They will simply not return. And you can imagine the "buzz" that will spread about this minor incident. It might sound something like this:

"Good polarity treatment, but the music was god-awful. It totally ruined the session for me." Why take the chance? It's always a good idea to have a few alternative CDs ready to use.

If you're unsure about the music, ask your clients if the music is to their taste or if they would prefer to listen to something else — or even prefer silence, in which to assimilate their experience — before you work on them.

The same holds true for incense. Not everyone enjoys it. In fact, I'd be very cautious about using it, especially the cone-shaped, colored kinds. They are very intense and some people have extreme adverse allergic reactions to the aroma or to the chemistry itself.

What noises are your clients listening to when they come to you for a treatment? If you work in a city, are there outside noises of traffic? Do you hear kids nearby yelling at each other? Is there a karate school above you? If any of these is a reality for you in your current office space, I suggest experimenting with ways to neutralize these distractions. These sounds can be very disturbing after even a short time and could make people feel edgy and uncomfortable. The people who come to you are paying you good money to help them, physically or mentally; they're also coming to you to relax. If you can't change the tone of the noise, you may want to ask the landlord for suggestions. Depending on his or her response, think seriously about moving or about making changes in your space to reduce the distractions.

A NIGHTMARE MASSAGE

I once had a massage in a woman's home where the space was worse than the most daunting nightmare. She escorted me into the back room of her house, where it was cold and damp. She had a candle burning with this awful scent that was much too strong and an incense stick smoking that was disgustingly sweet. She had a scratchy tape playing in the machine and her husband's TV was blaring from the next room. Had I not needed a massage so badly, I'd have gotten up from the table and told her that the environment was not conducive for me to relax. But I was too tired to move. I bit my lip through the entire massage and endured it. Never will I do that again.

Think about what *you'd* like when you go for a massage. What are the scents and sounds you enjoy smelling and listening to while you're lying down?

There are only a few places where I've felt totally relaxed, one-hundred-percent secure and at peace while receiving a treatment. One of these places is at my friend Aine Cafferty's house. My dear friend Aine is an exceptional Reiki practitioner and aromatherapist in Westchester, New York. The reason I feel so relaxed in Aine's space is not because she has expensive furniture or because she has high ceilings and a sophisticated stereo system. She lives in a modest studio apartment with wonderful big windows that provide lots of light. The colors in her apartment are soft and calming and she fills her space with lovely music, beeswax candles, flowers, plants, and a small waterfall — all adding to the soothing effect her place emanates. She gives one hundred and fifty percent of herself while she becomes the channel for the healing energy imparted by her Reiki masters to work through her. The woman is more dedicated to serving her clients than anyone I know, and it is for this reason that I've dedicated my book to her. Besides being an exemplary role model for the healing profession, she is filled with compassion and resonates with a poised gentleness.

YOUR PSYCHIC SPACE

Besides the physical space you create, there is the subliminal, but tangible, psychic space.

I went to see a chiropractor not too long ago. For the sake of confidentiality, I will call this man Mike. Mike was a very nice man, very sensitive, and had a very compassionate nature. He had a wonderful aura about him and I immediately felt relaxed in his presence. Now, I have been to many healers and I have always been aware of the energy field they create when they begin to work. I am able to feel it in their hands, in their voice, and in their silence while they are working with me. For some reason, perhaps because I was in the middle of writing this book, I became acutely aware of Mike's energy field the day I went to see him.

Allow me to draw you a clearer picture: I lay down on the table and Mike began to work on me. After only a few minutes, he stepped away to change the tape in his machine. The instant he moved out of the energy field that he'd created, the healing energy disappeared. The further he moved away from me, the colder I became, the less protected I felt. When he returned to my body, I'm sure he thought he would just continue where he'd left off. But it was not the same experience for me. It took several minutes before that supporting, healing energy returned.

When he left me again, this time to answer the door — it was a Federal Express man with a package — the same thing occurred. Only this time when Mike came back, it took even longer for me to feel embraced by the nurturing energy.

I believe what happened was that I felt subliminally abandoned. To some extent, it seems the healing energy field that is generated had a relational aspect to it. Now, who knows, this could stem from my own issue with abandonment. But when I've spoken to other practitioners about this issue and with friends who seek out healing sessions, they've understood immediately what I was talking about. I realized this is something that normally does not get verbalized. And because this was not an isolated experience, I began to speak to other practitioners about this issue.

What practitioners have explained to me is the following:

Regardless of the kind of healing the practitioner performs, he or she must first create a strong connection between himself or herself and the client. If there is the necessity to pause for the healing to take place or the practitioner needs to move around the table to work on another part of the body, there is still an energetic bond between the practitioner and the client. If the practitioner has done his or her own inner work, the integration should remain intact and the client should not feel abandoned.

If you are the only practitioner in your office and you are expecting deliveries, arrange for someone to come in and support you. Request that they answer the phone, the door, adjust the music. Find an assistant, a secretary or an intern to help you in these instances. Be attentive and conscious of the energy you create while you're working with your client. The healing that takes place is so subtle, so profound, why would you want to sabotage your efforts?

But, you may say, I'm just starting, working from a spare room in my house while my kids are in school, or I'm just doing this part time until I build my practice. Do the best you can. Leave a note on the outside door: "Please do not disturb until such-and-such a time." Put your answering machine on and place it in another room, so if it rings, it doesn't disrupt the session.

THE INNER CONNECTION

I was at a networking event not too long ago. People were chatting, the band was playing, couples were dancing — and there was this lady performing chair massages at the back of the room, massaging people's backs and necks. I watched her carefully as she moved around the chair and her client. She looked so intent on making her ten-minute client feel comfortable amidst all the chaos. I decided to sign up for a massage and was amazed to experience that even when her hands left my body to reach for the bottle of lotion, I could feel her energy connect with my subtle body. All the while the music was blaring and people were talking loudly, she remained intensely bonded with me, the person she was working on. I was so impressed with her that night that I signed up for several full-body sessions and have enjoyed every one of them.

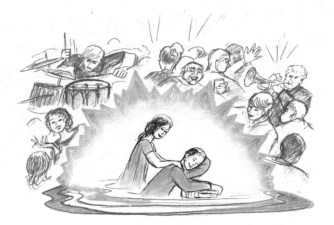

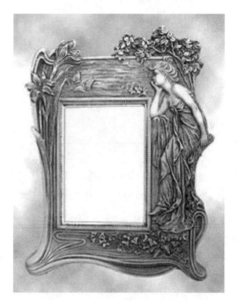

CHAPTER 5

CONCEIVING YOUR IDENTITY

Conceiving Your Identity

The direction of change to seek is not in our four dimensions:
it is getting deeper into what you are, where you are.

~ Thaddeas Golas,
Lazy Man's Guide to Enlightenment

This is the part of the book where you will need to dive deep inside yourself and answer questions that may not be so close to the surface. This is the time for contemplation, a time for searching your memory to recollect jobs and experiences you've had in the past. In some cases, this is where you will need to think back as to why you decided to go into the healing profession in the first place.

Whether you are transitioning from one career to another, just graduating from a certification curriculum or studies at a healing center, or wanting to expand your current practice, know that the strategy you will be creating for yourself will prove to be a reflection of how you relate to the world — and consequently, how the world reflects back to you. As the Bible states, "What ye sow, so shall ye reap." This is true for any profession. But especially true for the holistic practitioner.

It is our *dharma* (a Sanskrit word for *right action*) to stay conscious, to be aware of our actions at all times — actions toward ourselves as well as toward others. Knowing, with full awareness, that when we maintain this understanding on a continuous basis we will draw people to us who reflect the same beliefs. As soon as we shift into this perception, the clients coming to us will also shift.

For example, if you start complaining about the clients you are attracting, or the lack thereof, you may want to check inside yourself first. Ask yourself: What is it I'm doing? What is it that I'm thinking that attracts these people to me, or pushes others away?

We only attract our mirrors; have you noticed? Therefore, if you want to change your external circumstances, change what's going on inside *yourself* first.

One of the ways we can create this change and understand on the deepest level what we have to offer is by seeing ourselves from another perspective, from an objective standpoint. When we look at our accomplishments in black and white, on a sheet of paper in front of us, we see with our own eyes the value of our own worth. This is why the resumé is the first essential ingredient to the potion of success we are about to brew.

And if you are an affiliate with a healing center, every person involved in the center should go through the process of creating a resumé.

THE RESUME

Your resumé is the first and most significant part of your marketing and PR strategy. And as with all new endeavors that we want to cultivate and nurture, to make last so that our efforts make a difference, we need to create a strong foundation to build on.

I'd like to make a small wager that most of you reading this book do not have a current resumé sitting inside your computer ready for continuous updates. Now, perhaps you thought you could get away without writing one because you've remained at the same sort of work for years or because you've been in private practice for so long that you thought you didn't need one anymore. Perhaps you've been too busy to sit down long enough to write one out, or you were simply too lazy. Whatever the excuse may be, place your laziness, your business, your ego and all the concepts you've ever had about doing this task in another room for the time being and read carefully.

There are two reasons why every practitioner should have this document. The first and most important reason is for yourself. Simply writing the resumé builds self-confidence. Having the resumé empowers you to move forward and take immediate action. When you sit down and begin to flash back on everything you've done, all the hours of training and studying, all the bodies or minds you've worked with, all the jobs you labored at to get to where you are today, you will get a glimpse of how much you have accomplished and how your unique background places you in a special place to serve and heal. Knowing you are distinctive, even among the myriad of healers there are in the world, gives you the strength to persevere in the face of seeming brick walls you may run into.

The other reason I suggest writing a resumé is because one day, when it is the furthest thing from your mind, someone will ask you for this document — and because timing is everything, if you don't have one to hand over or send to this inquirer, you could lose the client or the opportunity for the position.

The fundamental bedrock for your practice is your resumé. If you do not have this piece of the marketing puzzle, please, do not wait another millisecond: go, get a piece of paper, a pen, and begin to write down all the jobs you've had within the past ten years (or the last five years, whichever you feel describes your background in the most positive light). Even if you've worked a job *pro bono* or helped out a friend and were not paid for that assignment, include it. You never know: that position you whimsically decided to accept at the last minute, for little or no money, because nothing else was going on in your life, may be the very job that lands you your next one.

After Samantha Williams, a Reiki practitioner, finished her resumé, she told me, "It was just like giving birth. I had to dig really deep into my past in order to remember all the experiences I had, and then I had to push them out, write them down. It was a long, painful labor. But after I did it, I felt twenty pounds lighter. I saw how much I had to offer people, how I had done things a little bit differently from other practitioners . . . The best thing," she went on, "was that I no longer had guilt about charging what I was worth."

MULTIPLE OCCUPATIONS

In case you happen to be an artist in addition to being a healer, or if you happen to be a chiropractor who is also a builder, please remember: *Do not include every job you've ever had in one resumé.* It will appear confusing to the reader. If you're a musician in addition to being a healer, do not list all your classical piano background on your "healing" resumé. It is best that you create a different resumé for each line of work that you participate in.

There was a time when I had three different resumés: a writing resumé, a PR/marketing resumé, and a theatrical resumé. On one occasion, I had to use all three in one week for different job applications. It felt really strange to hand out three different resumés. It was like I had multiple personalities. And yet, I had to admit these were all talents of mine — all marketable. When I was offered two out of the three jobs, I was glad I had moved through my limited understanding. From that day forward, I never felt weird handing out my diverse resumés again. Besides, once you've created one, it is very easy to create the second and the third.

EXPERIENCE THE EXPANSION

When you have completed writing down every job (within a five- to ten-year period), try to remember the dates you worked at each job. Place them before the name of the organization. Take the list over to your computer and input the data, fine-tune the language, spell-check all the words and then sit back and enjoy what you have created. You may be pleasantly surprised by the feelings that arise. Most likely, you will feel quite proud of yourself. You may experience an overwhelming sense of achievement, amazed at how much you have accomplished these past few years. This is exactly why the resumé is the first step toward building your foundation. It makes you feel good about you and all that you have accomplished.

I recall feeling so expanded after updating my resumé that when I went on an interview and handed my hot-off-the-press resumé to the prospective client, she said she didn't need to see it. I sat there in shock. I'd worked so hard and spent so much time and effort putting this thing together, why wasn't she interested? Only afterwards did she tell me that she sensed my confidence and ability to complete the tasks she'd called me in to do. I was especially blown away when she hired me for the job — on the spot.

You never know when you'll need this document. Every time you do a job, if it is relevant, place it on your resumé. Have the document ready and current, so you're able to print it out at a moment's notice. Then, you'll never have to say the words "Um, sorry, I, uh, don't have one."

SAMPLE RESUMES

Whether you're just starting your practice or you've had years of experience, you should be able to utilize at least one of the three resumés I've provided for you as examples. Please study each of them carefully, as they will help you to tailor your presentation of your own unique talents and experience.

The reason I chose these particular resumés is that each of them exemplifies a kind of clarity, professionalism and simplicity that many resumés do not. None of these three healers has crowded the page with excess words. They have not confused the reader by including other talents and skills. You will only see statistics that apply to the healing profession. These practitioners have only listed the necessities: healing certifications, dates, training and field experience.

Take your time, read them over. Feel free to use any one of them as a template. Adapt the style that best suits you, the one you have the most in common with, and then make it your own.

RESUME I: JUST STARTING OUT

Linda Frank is an art therapist from Santa Fe, New Mexico. I liked Linda's simple, up-front format. Her resumé is shorter than the other two, mainly because she hasn't had as much experience. However, I'm sure by the time this book reaches your hands, she will have had a few more jobs to include. The amount of employment is not what we are focusing on here; we are concerned with the form.

For those of you who have just graduated from a healing curriculum, Linda's resumé may be the perfect one for you to use as a model. Linda's resumé appears on the following page.

LINDA FRANK

ART THERAPIST

3749A State Highway 14, Santa Fe, NM 87508
505-473-9011; email: lindasfrank@hotmail.com

OBJECTIVE: Working with the elderly and developmentally disabled

EDUCATION:

Master of Arts in Art Therapy, Southwestern College, Santa Fe, New Mexico (October 2002)
University of Alabama at Huntsville, completing the prerequisites to enter the master's program at Southwestern; deans list (2000)
Masters degree in International Management, American Graduate School of International Management, Glendale, Arizona (1980)
Bachelor of Arts, Psychology and Spanish, University of New Mexico, Albuquerque, New Mexico (1978)
Junior year abroad; Knox College/Universidad de Barcelona, Spain (1976-1977)

FIELD EXPERIENCE:

Santa Fe Family Center, Santa Fe New Mexico
Art therapy intern, November 2001- September 2002
  • Individual and group art and play therapy.
Santa Maria el Mirador, Santa Fe, New Mexico
Art therapy intern, July 2002 - September 2002
  • Art therapy with two developmentally disabled individuals.
Sierra Vista, Santa Fe, New Mexico
Art therapy intern, July 2002 - September 2002
  • Art therapy with Alzheimer's patients in a residential setting.
Open Hands, Santa Fe, New Mexico
Art therapy intern, August 2002 - September 2002
  • An open studio environment doing art in an adult day facility serving the elderly and disabled.
Hands On Community Art, Santa Fe, New Mexico
Art therapy intern, September 2002 and July September 2001
  • An open studio environment doing art serving children and adults in the community.

Neaves Davis Detention Center, Huntsville, Alabama
Art therapy with adolescents, June - August 2000
   • Activities included facilitating an art group and a dream group.

PREVIOUS EXPERIENCE:

AMERICAN EXPRESS FINANCIAL ADVISORS, Huntsville, Alabama, 1994 - 1999
As an independent licensed personal advisor, responsibilities included developing
and implementing financial analysis and products for individuals and businesses. Areas of
specialization included protection planning, wealth accumulation, tax management,
retirement planning, and estate planning. Activities included interviewing clients about
their goals and financial situation. I established relationships with clients based on trust
and confidentiality.

ABANDACO INC, Manhasset, NY, and Decatur, Alabama, 1981 - 1992
Government Sales Manager, Responsible for government contracts. Developed and
implemented procedures for the management of subcontracts. Implemented quality assurance program that complied with government specifications.
Traffic Manager; Responsible for arranging both domestic and international trailer-load
and containerized shipments.

Additional Education:
Sand Play Training, 37 hours specialized training through Southwestern College and Sand
Play Therapists of America
Gestalt Training, 27 hours specialized training through Southwestern College and the
Gestalt Institute of Santa Fe

LANGUAGES: Spanish (fluent), Portuguese (working knowledge)

PROFESSIONAL AFFILIATION: American Art Therapy Association

References: Available upon request

RESUME 2: MORE ADVANCED

Joanne Ehret is a successful, sought-after acupuncturist in the New England area. Initially a graduate of the Swedish Institute, Joanne has studied in Beijing, China, and currently presents seminars up and down the East Coast. Joanne has been in private practice for over eighteen years. I met her several years ago when I had the privilege of representing her. I always admired and appreciated Joanne's strong business ethic, as she is one of those rare healers who truly understands the fine line between being a healer and being a businessperson (more about her holistic approach to business in ensuing chapters).

Joanne uses her curriculum vitae to show her certifications and training background and gives it only to clients who are interested in knowing more about her background, or to the media when they ask for it.

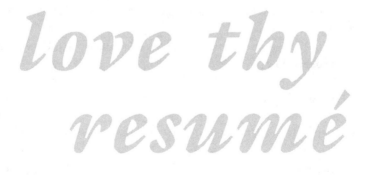

Joanne Ehret

Lic. Ac., D. Ac., Dipl. Ac., Dipl. C.H. (NCCA)

Chinese Medicine · Acupuncture · Gynecology, Internal Medicine and Pediatrics

53 Gothic Street · Northampton, MA 01060 · tel/fax (413) 586-9594

Professional Biography

Professional Experience

Private practitioner of Chinese medicine, Northampton, MA, 1983 to present

Professional translator of Chinese medical research journal articles, Blue Poppy Press, Boulder CO, 1999 to present

Classroom instructor and clinical supervisor of student interns, Tri-State Institute of Traditional Acupuncture, Stamford, CT, 1984 - 94

Education

Program in Chinese Medical Pediatrics, Blue Poppy Seminars, Boulder, CO, 1997-98

Program in Chinese Medical Gynecology, Blue Poppy Seminars, Boulder, CO, 1995-97

Clinical internship, Gynecology Outpatient Department, Xi Yuan Hospital of the China Academy of Traditional Chinese Medicine, Beijing, China, 1991, 81 hours

Program in Kanpo Yaku system of Chinese herbal medicine, New England School of Acupuncture, Boston, MA, 1988 - 90, 93 hours

Classroom study and clinical internship, Internal Medicine and Gynecology Departments, Xi Yan Hospital, Beijing, China, 1987, 200 hours

Program in Acupuncture, Tri-State Institute of Traditional Chinese Acupuncture, Stamford, CT, 1981 - 83

Program in Massage Therapy, Swedish Institute, New York, NY, 1978

Bachelor of Science in Environmental Education and Biology, Secondary Teaching Certificate, University of Michigan, Ann Arbor, MI, 1976

Licenses, Diplomas, Professional Memberships

Massachusetts License in Acupuncture

New York State License in Massage Therapy

Diplomate in Acupuncture and Chinese Herbal Medicine, National Commission for the Certification of Acupuncturists

Diplomate in Acupuncture, Tri-State Institute of Traditional Chinese Acupuncture

Fellow of the National Academy of Acupuncture and Oriental Medicine

RESUME 3: MORE COMPLEX

Clifford Shulman has been working with therapeutic movement and bodywork for over twenty years. Cliff's resumé is more complex than the others, as he has had a diverse range of training and experience. While Cliff has a thriving practice of his own, he enjoys working with other practitioners in therapeutic settings. He constantly updates his resumé, he told me, because if he is applying for a position in a facility (for instance Sloan-Kettering Institute), or at another physical-therapy clinic, he needs to have a current version immediately available.

Cliff placed his education at the beginning of his resumé. This works if you have a substantial amount to reveal in this category, as it makes an immediately impressive statement. If you do not have a strong list, I'd suggest placing this information at the end of the resumé.

Although Cliff also has a background in dance, you will notice that he has chosen to focus this resumé on his experience in therapeutic settings.

The resumé
builds self-confidence.
It empowers you
& reminds you
of all your past efforts.

CLIFFORD SHULMAN, P.T., C.T.P.

125 West 72nd Street, Suite 3F, New York, NY 10023
email address: marvelone@earthlink.net   (212) 712-2006

EDUCATION:
State University of New York, Stony Brook (BS in Physical Therapy, 1998)
Connecticut College (MA in Dance, emphasis in movement therapies, 1989)
The Boston Conservatory (BFA in Dance, 1975)

LICENSES:
Physical Therapist, New York State licensure, 1998
TRAGER® Practitioner, certified by The Trager Institute, 1990
Reiki Practitioner, certified by Usui shiki Ryoho, 1994

CLINICAL EXPERIENCE:
Over twenty years experience in the field of movement education, health and wellness. Using holistic approaches, physiotherapy, and mind-body education to provide an integrative approach to patient care.

• Private practice in Integrative Physical Therapy, integrating manual therapies (including Trager work, Myofascial release, Craniosacral therapy and Muscle Energy Technique methods), therapeutic movement and exercise, imagery and awareness into traditional treatment approaches. Work with individauls and groups to improve musculoskeletal, neurological, and stress-related conditions. Since 1998, New York, NY.

• St. Charles Rehabilitation Network, Albertson, NY. Clinical affiliation working with patients with neurological and orthopedic disorders. 05/98 - 07/98.

• West Side Dance Physical Therapy, New York, NY. Clinical affiliation working with patients with orthopedic problems, particularly performing artists (dancers, musicians). 12/97 - 3/98.

• Cabrini Medical Center, New York, NY. Clinical affiliation working with patients in acute care and short-term rehabilitation for orthopedic and neurological disorders. 06/97 - 08/97.

• Trager Pactitioner employed in the office of Dr. Christine Benner, DC. New York, NY, 1993.

• Private practice as Certified Trager Practitioner, New York, NY. Since 1991.

TEACHING EXPERIENCE:
Teaching experiential seminars in the uses of movement, imagery, touch, breath, awareness and meditation to groups.

• Memorial Sloan-Kettering Cancer Center's Integrative Medicine Service, New York, NY. Teaching class for outpatients and staff. Winter, 1999.

• Educational support staff for The Trager Institute, teaching Trager Mentastics Self-Care Movement Education and Introductory Workshop Leader since 1993.

• Produced Introductory videotape on The Trager Approach for The Trager Institute, 1996.

- Lincoln Center Institute, New York, NY. Led staff development programs and National Educator Workshops for teachers in the use of movement and inquiry-based learning approaches in the classroom.

- Faculty Appointments in Dance Movement Education:
  Princeton University, Princeton, NJ, Faculty, 1994-95.
  The Juilliard School, New York, NY, Faculty, 1992-94.
  Interlochen Center for the Arts, Interlochen, MI, Guest Faculty, 1988-89.
  Connecticut College, New London, CT, Guest Faculty, 1987.
  Florida State University, Tallahassee, FL, Visiting Asst. Professor, 198-83.

LECTURES AND DEMONSTRATIONS:

Presented lectures and demonstrations on The Trager Approach and mind-body approaches to healing, exercise and movement education in numerous locations, including:

4th Annual Int'l. Congress on Alternative & Complementary Therapies (DC)
The Arthritis Foundation (NY)
Gilda's Club for Cancer Patients (NY)
Beth Israel Medical Center P.T. Dept. (NY)
New York Open Center (NY)
Cabrini Medical Center P.T. Dept. (NY)
Jewish Home & Hospital (NY)
West Side Dance Physical Therapy (NY)
New Life Health Expo (NY)
Stony Brook University (NY)

RESEARCH:

- Investigated the relationship between movement therapies and creative problem-solving. Masters thesis, Connecticut College, 1989.

- Movement specialist researching development of visual-spatial learning in children, partnership of University of Nebraska/AAB and First Plymouth Preschool, 1999.

POST-GRADUATE STUDY:

- Extensive study of movement therapies including Trager Approach, Alexander Technique, Feldenkreis Method, Ideokinetic Facilitation, Laban Movement Analysis, and Bartenieff Fundamentals.

- Additional training in Manual therapies including Trager Approach, Myofascial release, Craniosacral therapy, Muscle Energy Technique, Proprioceptive Neuromuscular Facilitation.

HONORS:

Award for Outstanding Achievement, SUNY-Stony Brook, 1998.
Men of Achievement, London, 1994.

ESTABLISH AN E-MAIL ADDRESS

All three resumés have an e-mail address printed below the phone number. This small gesture indicates to employers and to clients that you are computer literate and have good business sense. And it makes it convenient for those who are on-line often to communicate with you effortlessly.

I am fully aware that some of you may not own a computer, nor want anything to do with one. You may also think that since the people coming to you for healing have complained about carpal tunnel, backaches, neck aches — all kinds of ailments resulting from the ongoing use of the computer — why in God's name would you want to start using the same machine that has created so much damage? Well, first of all, your job does not dictate that you use a computer as often as, let's say, a programmer or a writer. Secondly, these people who are spending all these hours at their desks, in front of their screens, will also be using their computers to find you, a practitioner who can heal their chronic ailments. Therefore, you may want to think seriously about establishing an e-mail address and (in the not so distant future) your own Website. (More on this topic in Chapter 9, Strategic Alliances and Internet Possibilities.)

THE BIO (BIOGRAPHY)

The biography is the second piece of groundwork to your foundation of outreach. Without one your journey could be bumpy, filled with unnecessary jolts that could slow you down or bring you to a halt in midstream. Why not go with the flow? Why not aim for smooth sailing and clear skies, unimpeded roads that make your journey graceful and enjoyable? There is absolutely nothing stopping you from moving through this next step with joy and excitement, is there?

Just remember, the mystery that is about to unfold will soon elevate you and your practice to an entirely new level. Stay focused. Read the chapters and paragraphs carefully. Take a deep breath and remember to practice and integrate. Practice and integrate.

The biography is similar to the resumé in that it provides background information regarding your professional experience. Nevertheless, it is a completely different animal. The bio is shorter, more cohesive, more personal than the resumé. The bio can also reveal interesting facts about you, facets that in most cases would be inappropriate to express on a resumé.

NOTE: It is much easier to establish your bio once your resumé has been fleshed out and finalized. So, do not even think about starting your bio until you've completed your resumé.

A bio is normally between one and three paragraphs long and can be used for various situations, including:

- When you are asked to be on a panel, and the sponsoring organization wants your bio to publicize you in the context of their event;
- For the media, to be attached to a press release, or to be included within a marketing packet;
- When a potential client wants to see an overview of your background.

There will be times when you will be asked for a shorter version — for example, for copy to be included in a brochure, or in a newspaper or magazine article. It's a good idea to have one long bio and one short one. I have included in this chapter the bios from the same people whose resumés we've seen in the previous pages. This way, you can see how each person has been able to transform his or her resumé into a solid, substantial biography.

Select the bio you most want to emulate and then return to the resumé from which it was derived. Notice how each of the practitioners has created a story about himself or herself by taking pertinent pieces of data from the resumé, and adding a small amount of personal background. This is not the time to write the novel or memoir you've thought about writing for years. It's about spicing up the relevant facts taken from your resumé, with a pinch of personal flavor. Be concise, as most potential readers only want to scan a couple of paragraphs.

As you reflect on writing your bio, become aware of any blocks you may have, any resistance, fears or insecurities that may come up. What are the voices in your head? Note any sensations, physically and energetically. Release them and then breathe. Release more of them and keep breathing deeply. Keep letting go. Remember what Lao-tzu said, "A journey of a thousand miles must begin with a single step." Keep this in mind as you look at and absorb the bios on the next few pages.

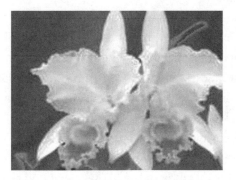

LINDA FRANK
Art Therapist
3749A Highway 14, Santa Fe, NM
Tel: 505 473-9011   E-mail: lindasfrank@hotmail.com

Linda Frank, a licensed mental-health counselor, holds a master's degree in art therapy from Southwestern College, Santa Fe, New Mexico. Her extensive internship experience in Santa Fe has included Open Hands, using art therapy with the elderly; Sierra Vista Retirement Community, an assisted-living facility, working with Alzheimer's patients; and Santa Maria el Mirador's day habilitation facility, working with individuals with developmental disabilities. While working as an intern at the Santa Fe Family Center, she used art and play therapy with children and with adults who had been abused.

Linda has received training from Southwestern College in sand play and in Gestalt techniques, as well as additional training through the Sand Play Therapists of America and the Gestalt Institute of Santa Fe.

After fulfilling her prerequisites for the master's program at the University of Huntsville in Huntsville, Alabama, Linda initiated and facilitated an art and dream group for adolescents at the Neaves Davis Detention Center. She also facilitated dream groups with the elderly and the homeless in Huntsville.

Linda Frank's intention is to use art as a catalyst to help individuals and groups experience transformation and empowerment, and manage transitions. Whether through visualization, active imagination or other transpersonal techniques, Linda believes that every individual has an artist within, and she works with individuals to encourage and awaken that artist and to validate the inner self.

Prior to her focus on art as therapy, Linda spent five years as a financial advisor for a Fortune 500 company. Her ability to honor confidentiality with clients and to be a team member allows her to work easily within an agency environment. Linda lives in Santa Fe, New Mexico. She is fluent in Spanish, and has a working knowledge of Portuguese.

JOANNE EHRET

Lic. Ac., D. Ac., Dipl. Ac. C.H. (NCCA)
Acupuncture and Chinese Herbal Medicine
53 Gothic Street, Northampton, MA 01060
Tel/fax (413) 586-9594   E-mail: jehret2@juno.com

Joanne Ehret is a licensed acupuncturist and national board certified in acupuncture and Chinese herbal medicine. She received her Bachelor of Science in Environmental Education and Biology and a secondary teaching certificate from the University of Michigan in 1976. After realizing her interests lay in health care, Ehret became a founding member of the Ann Arbor Women's Health Collective. In 1978 Ehret graduated the Swedish Institute of Massage as a licensed massage therapist while assisting at the Chelsea Neighborhood Clinic and the Chelsea Women's Health Team.

Ehret went on to study Chinese, Japanese, and European styles of acupuncture after learning of the body's vast network of meridians, the acupuncture energy channels. Learning that energetic change anticipates organic change, and that superior health care involves effective intervention at the energetic level to prevent or reverse the process of disease, Ehret knew what she wanted to do with the rest of her life.

In 1983 Ehret graduated the Tri-State Institute of Traditional Chinese Acupuncture in Stamford, Connecticut, and continued her studies at Xi Yuan Hospital in Beijing and at the hospital's advanced clinical course in Chinese medicine in 1987, where she completed advanced coursework in gynecology, digestive and respiratory systems, geriatrics, cardiology and neurology. In 1991, Ehret returned to the Xi Yuan Hospital in Beijing for further concentration in gynecology.

Currently based in Belchertown, Massachusetts, Ehret lectures and teaches in hospitals and health-care facilities throughout the United States. She has published several articles on acupuncture and Chinese herbal medicine and has appeared on national radio and TV shows. Ms. Ehret maintains a private practice in Northampton, Massachusetts, where she specializes in internal medicine, specifically respiratory, digestive, and gynecological disorders. Her clinic pharmacy contains over 300 individual herbs and formulas in tabulated, granule and tincture forms.

CLIFFORD SHULMAN, PT, CTP

125 W.est 72nd Street, Suite 3F, New York, NY 10023
Tel: 212 712 2006   E-mail: marvelone@earthlink.net

Clifford Shulman, PT, CTP is a licensed physical therapist and certified TRAGER® practitioner with a private practice in integrative physiotherapy. His practice integrates complementary therapies such as the Trager approach, myofascial release and craniosacral therapy, therapeutic movement, guided imagery and mind-body approaches to the treatment of chronic pain and dysfunction. He first began working with holistic approaches to movement reeducation, health and wellness in the late 1970s and was certified in the method developed by Milton Trager, M.D., in 1990. He is on the educational support staff of the Trager Institute, for whom he has also produced an introductory videotape. He was interviewed by Carol Martin on the national cable television program, *Alive and Wellness.*

A respected educator as well as therapist, Mr. Shulman has presented lectures on a mind-body approach to exercise to the Arthritis Foundation and Gilda's Club New York, and has taught a class for recovering cancer patients at the Integrative Medicine Center of Memorial Sloan-Kettering Cancer Center in New York. Mr. Shulman has also led lectures and demonstrations of his approach in numerous other forums, including the Fourth International Conference on Complementary and Alternative Therapies, Beth Israel Medical Center Physical Therapy Department, Cabrini Medical Center, West Side Dance Physical Therapy, Stony Brook University, New York Open Center and others.

Long interested in facilitating greater movement potential and awareness in people of all ages, Mr. Shulman has also been active in teaching educators how to introduce movement into classroom studies and recently led a National Educators Workshop for Lincoln Center Institute.

For those occasions when a shorter bio is necessary, here is a condensed version of Cliff's resumé.

CLIFFORD SHULMAN, PT, CTP

125 West 72nd Street, Suite 3F, New York, NY 10023
Tel: 212 712 2006   E-mail: marvelone@earthlink.net

Clifford Shulman, PT, CTP is a licensed physical therapist and certified TRAGER® practitioner with a private practice in integrative
physiotherapy in New York. His practice integrates complementary
manual therapies, therapeutic movement, exercise and mind-body
approaches in the treatment of musculoskeletal, neurological and
chronic pain disorders. A respected educator as well as therapist,
he has led workshops and seminars on innovative approaches to
movement, exercise and healing for numerous audiences, including
the Arthritis Foundation, Gilda's Club, Memorial Sloan-Kettering
Cancer Center, and the Fourth International Conference on
Complementary and Alternative Therapies. He is on the educational
support staff for the Trager Institute, for whom he has produced an
introductory videotape and teaches introductory workshops and
Trager Mentastics movement education.

THE SOUND BITE

Believe it or not, the first ten seconds of your in-person self-introduction tells more about you than you could ever imagine. In those first few seconds, the person you are talking to hears the sound of your voice, the tone of your voice. They see, and even feel, your body language. They see how you hold yourself, how secure you are. They see if and how you make eye contact. They get a sense of whether or not they can trust you or if they feel comfortable in your presence.

Isn't this true for *you*? When someone walks into a room, do you not automatically form an opinion about them? When someone walks into your office or calls you on the telephone for the first time, don't you make spontaneous conclusions? Trust me, you do; we all do, and usually within the first ten seconds. Hundreds of books have been written about "the first impression," "the first glance," "the first sentence." Knowing this to be true, I tried a little experiment with a few audience members at a workshop I led in New York City.

The audience was filled with a diverse crowd of practitioners. I asked if five men and five women would please volunteer for a game. Ten practitioners raised their hands and came to the front of the room. I told them: "Let's pretend we are at a networking brunch. I'm going to come up to each one of you and introduce myself and then you are to introduce yourself to me."

I went up to the first person and said, "Hi, my name is Andrea Adler. I'm a PR/marketing consultant specializing in the holistic industry. I offer private consultations, representation, and workshops, and have recently written a book called *Creating an Abundant Practice: A Spiritual and Practical Guide for Holistic Practitioners and Healing Centers*. What do you do?"

After each practitioner introduced himself or herself, the audience was stunned to see that only one out of ten people had actually articulated in less than four sentences what he or she did for a living. Three out of the ten practitioners rambled on and on without being definitive, others stumbled and tried to remember what it was they'd written on their brochure. One man pulled out his card and read it out loud. A woman in her forties stated enthusiastically, "I'm a massage therapist. I work on people's bodies," which was a truthful statement but not very informative or imaginative.

Seeing this, I developed a way in which practitioners can move out of their mental constructs about who they are and how they present themselves. I now spend an hour to an hour and a half introducing improvisational theater exercises into my workshops. Through these games, practitioners learn to act and react from a place of strength and confidence. The games become a catalyst for letting go of outdated habits, guards, and inhibitions as they explore new ways to present themselves. As a result, participants become more agile and flexible. They begin to trust instinctively how to articulate who they are, and their sound bite comes to them without struggle.

Practitioners are not the only professionals who have difficulty explaining to others what they do. Lawyers, artists, manufacturers, designers, businessmen, all experience this awkwardness — and most of them have no idea that their presentation, or lack thereof, can make or break a relationship, block people from coming to their door, obstruct the potential of a flourishing business, set limits on the good that they can offer others.

I cannot emphasize enough the significance of having these words, your *sound bite,* be compelling and powerful, memorized and flowing effortlessly from your lips.

The sound bite conveys to people the essence of what you do. It consists of two to four lines that describe in detail who you are and what your specific modality is. The sound bite is a teaser. It whets your hearers' appetites. Attract them, get their attention, and they'll want to learn more. If your words are effective, the listener will be so intrigued by what you say that he or she will want to set up an appointment and try out this method you have spoken so fascinatingly about.

Professionals who are truly successful know how necessary it is to have this aspect of their presentation down pat. They do not waver in their ability to articulate who they are and what they can do for you. They get right to the point and don't waste your time.

Because there will always be diverse audiences you will be speaking to, it would be useful for you to have two or three variations on the tip of your tongue:

- For the person who has never heard of your technique before;
- For the person who is a practitioner in another field and has a little knowledge of your technique;
- For the peer who has a lot of knowledge, but needs to understand how you are unique.

Cliff Shulman uses the following sound bites when he is speaking to people about the Trager technique. This is how he varies the information:

If he is talking to a person who has never heard of Trager before, he will say:

Trager is a type of bodywork that relieves deep-seated physical restrictions and pain. By using a combination of gentle touch and rhythmic movements, it increases mobility and reduces stress.

If he is talking to another therapist, he will say:

Trager is a type of bodywork and movement reeducation that relieves deep-seated physical restrictions and pain. It increases mobility and reduces stress through a combination of gentle touch, rhythmic movement and awareness. Developed by Dr. Milton Trager, a doctor of physical medicine and rehab, it's been effective in helping people with a variety of conditions, both musculoskeletal and neurological.

If he is talking to a doctor, he will say:

Trager is a form of movement reeducation developed by Dr. Milton Trager that involves both passive and active motion to facilitate the release of deep-seated restrictions. It creates change through engaging the sensory-motor feedback loops and is extremely helpful in relieving muscle guarding, pain, and rigidity in patients due to musculoskeletal pain as well as to certain neurological disorders.

If they want more information, he'll add:

The practitioner employs a variety of rhythmic oscillations that are profoundly relaxing to the nervous system while guiding the individual through range of motion and movements such as rocking, swinging, shaking or tractioning.

This is an exercise I use in my workshops. You may want to try it for coming up with your sound bites:

1. Close your eyes and contemplate what it is you want to convey.

2. Try to create a sensory impression. Find words that conjure up images and create a picture in the listener's mind. Play with words that evoke excitement and delight, interest and intrigue.

3. When you are ready, write down a few sentences. Keep coming up with different phrases until you are satisfied with two or three of them.

4. Speak into a tape recorder and listen to how these words sound to you. Keep exploring diverse ways of interpreting who you are.

5. When you have come up with a few options, go out and testmarket them. Repeat them to friends and ask them which ones they like the best. Try them on people you don't know.

Don't give up. There's a quality that you're looking for that can be shared with people which reveals your enthusiasm. These words will come to you in time, I promise.

Take note of how friends and strangers react to your sound bite. Did they look confused, or did they get it right away? Did they want or need more information? Did they look interested and *want* more information, or did they look confused and *need* more information? All these reactions will take you closer to finding the phrasing that is perfect for you.

By having your sound bite firmly committed to memory and in the forefront of your brain, you will never have to experience the embarrassment of wavering or stumbling as you describe to potential clients or to the media who you are and what your particular practice is about.

Use the space on the next page to write down your sample sound bites:

To a person who has never heard of your method:

_____
_____
_____
_____
_____
_____

To another practitioner:

_____
_____
_____
_____
_____
_____

To a peer:

_____
_____
_____
_____
_____
_____

Besides having your sound bite memorized and ready for your delivery, don't forget to smile. When you genuinely smile, you radiate friendliness and interest in others. Your smile conveys a feeling of warmth and openness, and inspires confidence. So, stand with confidence, speak with confidence, and smile with confidence.

YOUR BUSINESS CARD AND BROCHURE

Congratulations! You have just laid the cornerstones of your foundation: creating wholeness, envisioning your future, completing your resumé, your bio and your sound bite. You should feel extremely proud of yourself. I suggest you treat yourself to a nice meal, call friends and invite them to dinner, call your massage therapist and schedule a massage, go to a spa. Do something that you truly enjoy, to reward yourself — you've earned it!

When you return from treating yourself, take a few minutes to ponder the next two items: your business card and your brochure. In case you do not have these in your possession, it is now time to think seriously about having them made up, as they are the next pieces of marketing collateral you will need on hand before you begin your outreach.

There are marketing materials and there are marketing materials. The ones that stand out, take hold of your senses, are usually the ones that people have taken the time to think about and create. They look and feel wonderful: the quality of the paper is substantial, the font is legible, the colors resonate with the subject matter. The text isn't crowded. But most importantly, the writing speaks to you. You are receiving the information you need to make an educated decision about whether to call the practitioner whose brochure or card you are reading.

THE CARD

If you think about it, conversation is air. Once your words are out there, in the universe, so to speak, they disappear, disintegrate into the ether. They can of course make a lasting impression — "the power of the word" we'll explore in Chapter 8 is one of my favorite topics — but that's only if the people you're talking to are listening carefully and comprehending your message.

Although your resumé and biographies are tangible pieces of collateral, you wouldn't hand either one of these pieces of paper to someone you've just met. You would leave them with your card.

You never know when you'll be sitting next to someone on the train, in a restaurant, at a friend's dinner party, who just may happen to need your service. When you have a card to hand to them, it subliminally creates trust. They see you have your act together — and most importantly, they have a way in which to contact you if they decide to call you for an appointment or for more information.

Whatever you do, even if you are watching your pennies, do not make up cards on the computer that are printed on regular paper stock. They are flimsy and in most cases do not hold up longer than a few days. And even pre-formed business-card stock available commercially often leaves bumpy edges where you've torn the perforations to produce your do-it-yourself cards. There's a ragged feel to these cards in the hands of a client — not the feeling of richness, assurance, that you want to convey. So unless you have high-quality card stock and a fabulously clean-cutting paper trimmer, go to a local printer and outsource your card supply.

A printer can create your business cards for as little as twenty or thirty dollars. Your cards don't have to be elaborate. They don't have to fold out or have raised lettering. You can keep the card very simple and inexpensive.

A card should include the following information:
- your name
- your title
- your modalities (if you use more than one)
- your phone and fax number
- your address
- your e-mail address
- your Website address (if you have one)

What I've seen on some business cards that adds a nice touch is placing your contact information on the front with a brief description of your service on the back. This small addition allows the recipient to look at the card at a later date and be provided with more particulars about you than simply reading *massage therapist.* You can also have a card that opens up and describes your modality inside. Just don't place too much information on the card. Keep it airy with a lot of white space between the text which allow the letters to be easily read.

According to *Grassroots Marketing:Getting Noticed in a Noisy World,* by Shel Horowitz, there are various kinds of cards that can be used. Here are a few that Shel Horowitz mentions:

The Fold-out

The fold-out card can be very impressive. It's like a mini-flyer. You can make it with one of the flaps smaller, so it is obvious to the reader that the card opens. Know that two-sided printing costs more, but it can make a difference in your presentation.

Rolodex

The Rolodex card is slightly bigger than the normal business card. It's a practical approach for those who keep a Rolodex file mounted on their desks. The fact that the cards fit nicely on the file, with a tab that sticks up, allows people to find your card easily.

If you are planning to create your own cards, Paper Direct **(800-272-7377)** sells Rolodex card stock. Otherwise, your local printer will have options to show you.

Rolodex Oversize

You might think you could get more information on one card, or that your card will stand out, if it's oversize. But these good intentions are negated by the fact that people have to jump hoops trying to store the card. If it doesn't fit into a card file, it's too big for the Rolodex. So what will happen is, they'll stuff the card into a drawer and forget about it.

Picture and Hologram Cards

Cards with photographs on them will certainly get noticed, but you will pay the price. Think hard before you place a photo on the card. Think about what you are wanting to convey to a prospective client. Perhaps the additional funds would be better spent on creating an outstanding logo.

As for hologram cards that shimmer when you move the card, you many want to ask yourself here, too: is it worth the price?

Magnetic Cards

Magnetic cards can be quite effective as an additional marketing tool. They become great reminders when people use them on their refrigerators to hold the family photo.

Here are a few of my favorite cards. The reason I like them is because they are intriguing, easy to read and contain all the essentials.

Holistic Psychotherapy

Ingrid Willgren, MA
support and guidance
through life's transitions

by appointment:
845. 353. 7384
Nyack, NY

DJUNA WOJTON

507 Fairmount Avenue
Philadelphia PA 19123
Tel 215 627.6710
Fax 215 922.1427
djunaverse@aol.com
www.djunaverse.com

Tarot | Astrology | Soul & Past Life Healings | REIKI

Spacial Harmony

"Opening Your Environment To Universal Harmony"

With
Feng Shui

Barbara
Certified Feng Shui Consultant
By Appointment Only

Phone/Fax: (914) 738-6032
Email: spclhrmony@aol.com
http//members.aol.com/spclhrmony

Denise Weber, MA

Body-Psychotherapy

203•544•6094

18 Samuelson Road
Weston, Connecticut 06883

THE BROCHURE

The brochure is another integral part of your campaign. It is something you will want to make hundreds of copies of and leave everywhere you think your audience will appear.

Paper, like information, spreads, and brochures especially get passed around by a lot of people. The person picking up the brochure may not need it for himself or herself, but may pass it on to friends and relatives who do. So, do not be frugal with your brochures: give them away, leave them in strategic places, pass them on to neighbors and friends, health-food stores.

I'm sure you've seen countless brochures throughout your life. Well, now is the time to take a closer look at these pieces of collateral. You know what it's like when you're purchasing a car — all of a sudden you begin to look at every car that drives down the street. You begin to notice the size of the bumper, the color of the car, the lines of the exterior, the headroom and elbowroom of the interior. Quite spontaneously, your antennas go up and you have a heightened awareness of cars you never had in the past.

Bring those antennas up now as you begin to study every brochure that crosses your path. Notice how some have a glossy finish, some have a matte finish. Some have warm color tones, others are bright and flashy and scream for your attention. There are brochures that have pictures on the cover or artwork inside. Some have a lot of text and others leave a lot of white space around the text. As you begin to study these brochures, become aware of the emotional reaction you have to each one. See which ones appeal to you and which do not, which draw you in and which repel you and push you away.

Creating your brochure is a delicate process that takes time and contemplation. Practitioners who have rushed with the creation of their brochure virtually never feel good with the end results. You want to feel proud when you hand someone your brochure. It is your calling card and an important piece of collateral that will express to people the heart of what you do.

The most important thing to remember is this:

Do not sit down and write what you think people should know about you and your practice. Instead, sit, meditate, ask yourself: What is it my potential clients would like to read on these pages that will educate them about who I am and what I have to offer? What are the words I should use that will draw these people to me?

I've provided an exercise that will help you get in touch with this process, get in touch with what you already know but at times feel blocked to channel. I call it "The Brochure Contemplation."

THE BROCHURE CONTEMPLATION

First, get a pencil and a blank piece of paper and fold it in a tri-fold, like a brochure.

Sit down on a chair near a table or move into a comfortable cross-legged posture on the floor. Place the folded piece of paper and the pencil in front of you.

Prepare yourself for meditation.

Take a deep breath in, and breathe out long. Take another deep breath, and breathe out long.

Allow yourself to be the channel for the information that you know so well to come through you with ease.

Ask yourself: What would my readers like to see on the front panel of this brochure? What should it say that will make them want to open it up and read more?

Take your time and allow yourself to see the words and the images, if any visuals arise, on the page.

When we write from the perspective of "What does my audience want to read that will provide them with the information, that will resonate with their hearts and minds?" rather than "This is what I want my readers to know," the brochure becomes a heartfelt message, rather than a series of didactic words that could turn readers off.

Is there an image or logo that comes up for you, that you would like to create? If so, begin to draw that image. Even if it's a rough draft. You can always refine it later.

Once you have a sense of what the front panel should look like, open the brochure and contemplate the second panel.

The second panel, the panel on the far left, should either explain what your modality is and what your practice is about (like a short mission statement), or it should be a letter by you to your audience. This panel, like the front panel, sets the tone for the rest of the brochure.

Once again, meditate on being the channel for this information to come through you.

The third and fourth panels should explain your modality(ies) in detail and how they can help the reader. Perhaps these panels are filled with descriptions of your services. These pages could also include a quote or two from someone who has benefited from your service.

The fifth panel can display your picture and your bio.

The sixth panel can either be used as a self-mailer or contain information on how your audience can reach you.

There is no set-in-stone way of creating a brochure. Let your imagination take charge and discover for yourself what your audience would like to see. Take your time, do not rush; allow your thoughts to come through unimpeded. Once you have a first draft, put it aside for a few hours, or even a few days. When you are in a fresh state with new eyes, take another look at what you designed and fine-tune it, edit out the inadequacies or flesh out the parts that need to be filled in.

Before you take your final draft to the printer or to the graphic designer, make sure you have several people read it. Several sets of eyeballs looking over your material is better than your two alone. No matter how many times we go over a draft, we can easily miss spelling and grammar mistakes, and even areas that are not clear or where the tone needs a subtle but important shift. Listen to what your readers say, see if it resonates with your intention, and make the appropriate changes.

GRAPHICS

Unless you are very clever with graphics and know how to place text on paper, I'd highly recommend that you contact a professional graphic designer to help you with the layout of your brochure. I have seen many brochures that look unprofessional because practitioners either were in a hurry and needed to have their brochures printed immediately or they couldn't afford to hire someone and they did it themselves.

If you can't afford to hire a graphic designer, perhaps you know a friend who is artistic and knows about layout. You may want to consider bartering. In either case, here are a few things to keep in mind:

- Leave as much white space around the text as possible. Don't clutter the brochure with too many words.
- Include your logo (if you have one) somewhere on the

brochure. An interesting logo draws attention to your brochure and can look quite attractive. When you've selected a logo that represents your practice, duplicate it on your cards, on your stationery, on your flyers and on all your marketing materials. Repetition works in this instance. People will begin to recognize your logo and associate it with you.

On the cover of my first book, I used the image of the eagle. I also used the eagle on all my marketing materials at that time. I used this image for several reasons: my last name, *Adler,* means *eagle* in German. And although I am not of German descent, I used the image because it conjures up soaring, flight, freedom, and fearlessness. That is what I've starved for in my own life and it is what I've wanted my clients and participants in my workshops to experience for themselves.

I have recently changed my logo and my entire expressive image. As I move into a whole new phase of my life, I am exploring the image of flowering, opening and expanding. I worked with a graphic designer for hours until we came up with an image that resonated with what my heart wanted to see on the page.

- A photo of yourself is a wonderful addition to your brochure. However, *where* you place your photo is extremely important. If you are an individual practitioner and want to include your picture, do not place it on the front cover. It draws too much attention to yourself, instead of to your service. The message you transmit to the public is: *I'm the star here. Come see me.* Is this what you want potential clients or partners to think? If you are creating a brochure for a healing center, it's a different story. In this case, presenting readers with the image of the staff or practitioners in your clinic is a nice touch. The message conveys to people: *We are all here to help you. We are caring, concerned practitioners. This is what we look like. You can trust us.* If you decide to feature your staff in a photo, they should look healthy, neat, caring and intelligent.

- Be sure to gather short testimonials from your satisfied clients. What other people say about you is many times more persuasive to readers than what you have to say about yourself.

I have selected a few brochures to highlight. Clearly, these practitioners had taken time to think about the images, the colors (even though all you see is black and white), and the words. They worked with professional graphic designers and, as a result, have in their possession stunning, professional marketing pieces to hand out.

Remember:

if your brochure looks cluttered and unprofessional, that will be the impression people will be left with. If your brochure looks intriguing, trim, and well thought out, that will be the impression people will walk away with. Which would you prefer?

Energy Balancing

We are made of energetic elements. From our foundation of atoms and molecules, to the intricate pathways that support our physiological functions, to the vibrant living force within us and surrounding us, energy is an integral part of our lives.

The harmonious flow of energy through the body ensures good health and well-being in body, mind, and spirit.

Stress, discomfort, trauma, or simply the complexities of daily life can challenge the smooth and proper circulation of energy. This is when energy bodywork can be of great assistance.

The beauty of this work is that it mirrors the way our body naturally heals and sustains itself. Energy bodywork can help restore balance, or bring us to a new place of balance, thereby renewing our vitality and inspiring us to move forward with steadiness and insight.

Results

Clients experience a broad range of results with energetic bodywork, from improvement in physical symptoms to greater enjoyment and appreciation of life.

Common Results include:

- Greater ease in functioning
- Decreased pain and discomfort
- Enhanced immunity
- Ability to field life's challenges
- Integration
- Alignment
- Centeredness
- Peace of Mind, Contentment
- Improved relationships with others
- Relaxation

Sessions last about 1 hour, and are received through comfortable clothing.

Miriam welcomes you as a client.

For an appointment or further information:

520.743.7577

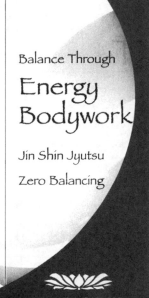

Balance Through

Energy Bodywork

Jin Shin Jyutsu

Zero Balancing

Miriam Bloomfield L.M.T.
520.743.7577

Jin Shin Jyutsu®

This physio-philosophy is an ancient art of harmonizing the flow of life energy in the body. Born of innate wisdom and passed down through the generations by word of mouth, it was dramatically revived in the early 1900's by Master Jiro Murai in Japan. After clearing himself of life-threatening illness, Master Murai devoted the rest of his life to the research and development of Jin Shin Jyutsu. The resulting knowledge was imparted to Mary Burmeister, who brought it to the United States in the 1950's.

Jin Shin Jyutsu employs 26 "safety locks" along energy pathways, which feed life into our bodies. When one or more paths become blocked, the resulting stagnation can disrupt the local area and eventually disharmonize the complete energy flow. Holding these energy locks in combination can return us to balance in body, mind and spirit.

Miriam Bloomfield L.M.T.
Energy Bodywork

Known as the "Art of Longevity" and the "Art of Happiness", Jin Shin Jyutsu facilitates our own profound healing capacity. Subtle, with deep, far-reaching effects, it may be utilized for any condition.

It is also a potent ally when applied as self-help. Self-help classes are available for individuals and groups.

Zero Balancing®

Zero Balancing is a simple yet powerful method of aligning body energy with the body's physical structure. Developed by Dr. Fritz Smith, a doctor of medicine, osteopathy and acupuncture, it embodies a profound understanding of both Eastern and Western traditions of healing.

The practitioner uses "fulcrums" or gentle pressure in foundational areas of holding, including the back, neck, hips and feet to create stronger, clearer fields of energy in the body/mind.

By aligning the densest tissues of the body (the bone and skeletal system) with the energy moving through them, Zero Balancing allows the release and dissolution of limiting and uncomfortable patterns of all kinds.

A renewed sense of integration, grounding, wholeness and balance can be experienced.

"In pursuing deeper understanding, I have experienced directly how energy sustains and balances us. The fruit of my experience is an ability to address each client's whole being through sensitive, informed touch."

— Miriam Bloomfield

Meet The Practitioner

Miriam graduated from Stanford University with a B.A in History. She began her studies as a Bodywork Practitioner and a student of meditation in 1982 and they continue to this day.

She graduated from the Swedish Institute of Massage in New York in 1986 and is a Licensed Massage Therapist in New York and Arizona. Miriam is a Certified Zero Balancing Practitioner and a Certified Practitioner of Jin Shin Jyutsu. She currently specializes in Energy Bodywork.

In addition to private practice, Miriam has been on staff at Chiropractic and Naturopathic Clinics, Wellness Centers, Health Clubs and Resorts.

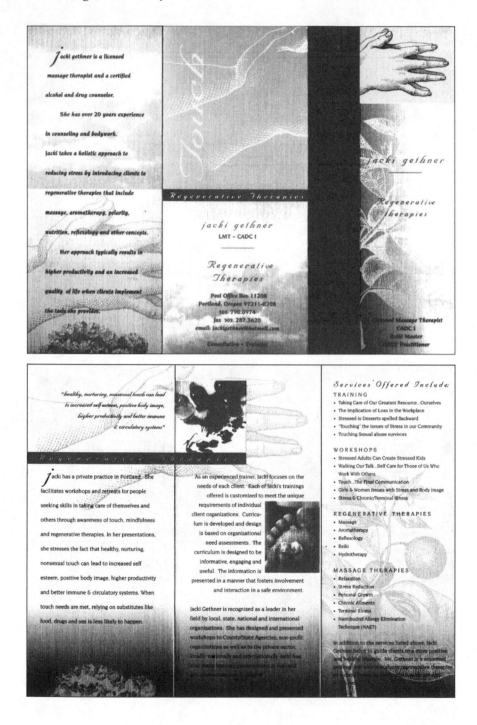

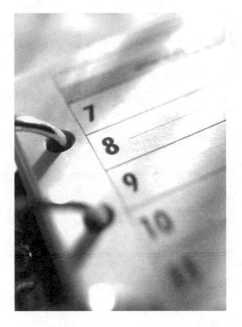

CHAPTER 6

EXPLORING
YOUR COMMITMENTS

Exploring Your Commitments

Know the white, yet keep the black. Be a pattern for the world;
the two will be strong inside you and there will be nothing you can't do.
~ Tao te Ching

Ahhh, to be able to wake up every morning and venture off to a job you absolutely love, earning your living doing what you cherish, what you've been gifted by God to share with others. To be able to tour the world, see exotic places and, at the same time, teach your healing method to others — all the while getting reimbursed by the IRS for your excursion. What a divine lifestyle. Sounds like a dream, doesn't it? There is no reason why this scenario can't manifest in your life next month, next year, in the next three to five years. It's not an unattainable goal — if that's your intention. By the way, what *is* your intention? What is your future? If it is to travel the world and teach or lecture, what steps do you need to take in order to get there?

The reality is, to have a fulfilling career in any industry, you need to evaluate where you are in your life right now, understand that the roles to which you are obligated today can help you plan your next move more realistically for tomorrow.

It begins with a few questions you ask yourself today. For example, if you are a wife and mother of two young children and you've recently graduated from massage school, there are some obvious limitations you're going to encounter in terms of how much time you can commit to developing your practice. If you are still a student, in school, you will need to think about how much time you can commit to working part-time as a healer, knowing the responsibility you have to studying and maintaining your good grades.

EXPLORING YOUR PARAMETERS

By answering the following questions, you will be able to determine how broad or how narrow a commitment — how many hours a day, how many hours a week — you can make to your practice or to your holistic career.

What is your family status? Are you a mother, a father, a wife, a husband, a caretaker, a landlord? Write down all your roles:

_____

_____

_____

_____

_____

Are you involved in any other business endeavors or community service? If so, how much time do you devote to them?

Commitment _____

Time devoted _____

Commitment _____

Time devoted _____

Commitment _____

Time devoted _____

You will need to think about the time it takes you to get from point A to point B. Do you have a car, or do you depend on public transportation?

_____

How far are you willing to travel to see a client or present a seminar?

_____

_____

Do you prefer working alone, or with other people?

_____

_____

Do you enjoy working in the house, or do you prefer an office setting?

_____

_____

Now, make an estimate of how many hours you could feasibly spend on your practice or your career for the next six months:

_____

_____

Consider asking yourself these questions every six months, as the answers will guide you and help you to determine how many hours a day or week you can devote to your marketing and PR outreach. Know that this time commitment will constantly change. As you take a close look at your boundaries, they will in the end give you tremendous freedom to pursue the dreams you intend for yourself.

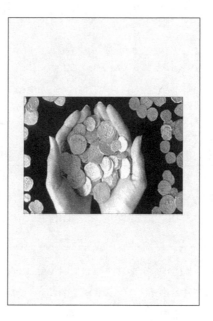

CHAPTER 7

GATHERING THE
GOLDEN NUGGETS

Gathering the Golden Nuggets

*As we begin to trust ourselves to move into new realms, we find
the courage to gather the golden nuggets that surround us.*

~ Andrea Adler

Now that you have completed the *Inner Journey* (at least in reference
to the purposes we are exploring in this book), and you are aware
of how many hours you can devote to your outreach, you are ready
to begin the process of gathering all the golden nuggets that surround you.

Isn't it interesting how at times we feel we have to look far beyond
our immediate surroundings to find "gold"? And yet, there are so
many precious opportunities so close to us that sometimes we can't
see them. It's one thing to have a vision of the future and see the
panorama of possibilities, it's another to be here now and not miss
the options that are right in front of us.

A few years ago I was in Florida presenting a keynote speech
and met a woman, a massage therapist, who asked if she could
have a consultation. I went to her home and she told me that
she'd wanted to build her practice in her house because she was
a single parent with two small children. She said she had made
several attempts to promote it, but all of her current clients preferred that she come to their homes for a massage. As she was talking to me, I sat on her porch looking directly across the street at

a strip mall. There was a bank, a beauty shop, a few restaurants, an office building and a dry cleaner's. I wondered if she had approached any of these establishments. When I asked her if she had, she said, "No, it never occurred to me to walk into any of those places." I couldn't believe the opportunities that were so close to her. By the end of the consultation, we had created a post-card and a flyer that offered the staff and the owners of these establishments one free massage for every three massages they signed up for.

LOOK AROUND YOU

If we were to just walk out our door and look around the corner, across the street, down the block, we would see how many opportunities there are right near us. It's when we try to look too far, achieve too much too soon, or move beyond our local surroundings before we've looked close by, that we end up becoming frustrated, talking ourselves into giving up — or worse, stopping. Step back, look at your immediate surroundings first, then branch out.

Here's another example: a friend of mine, Sally, a Qigong thera-pist and a registered nurse, had just moved to Tucson, Arizona from Connecticut. She had gone through a messy divorce and wanted with all her heart to have a home of her own. She was fifty-seven, and found a lovely, affordable two-bedroom ranch in a retirement com-munity just outside Tucson.

She immediately began to drive forty miles every day, back and forth to Tucson, looking for Qigong opportunities. When I came for a short visit, she was beside herself and ready to give up. She was frus-trated and upset, sure she'd made the wrong purchase — living in a community where the average age was seventy-four.

After only a few days of scouting out the area, I couldn't believe that she hadn't seen the opportunities that were, literally, all around her. Not only were there well-to-do retirees in every house, on every block of her housing development for miles. These people were well educated. They cared about their health. They joined local gyms and took walks every day. They clearly wanted to live as long as possible in a healthy body.

Perhaps they'd never had the time to explore complementary medicine while they were working and planning for their retirement. Perhaps they had heard about Qigong, but were too busy to learn more about it. If either of these scenarios were the case, they certainly had time now.

Surrounding the neighborhood were four recreational centers that 90 percent of the homeowners participated in. These centers offered crafts and sports, educational programs, gardening tips. All my friend had to do was work part-time as an RN to keep the money flowing as she built her practice, and offer introductory programs on Qigong at all four centers. She could even offer house calls — a thing of the past, but a benefit most people still appreciated, especially these people. She could, if she were so inclined, open an office or rent out space from a nearby clinic.

This was a huge opportunity for my friend, as well as for her new community. Why not at least see if Qigong would be something her new neighbors would like to experiment with and include in their maintenance program? I can't wait to hear how the magic begins to work, once she starts these intro programs. She promised to keep me updated.

START WHERE YOU ARE

We can always move into other communities, other cities, other states, later. Obviously, if we live in a place like Manhattan, we'll have more of a selection than someone who lives in Hurleyville, a small hamlet in upstate New York. However, the advantage of living in a small town is that there's always the next town — and the next. There will always be the occasion to expand geographically.

To get a jump-start on where to look, please answer the following questions and fill in each blank with as many specifics as possible:

What geographical location do you live in?

_____

_____

_____

What big cities are close by?

_____

_____

_____

What small cities or towns are close by?

_____

_____

_____

What kinds of people surround you? Blue-collar, white-collar? Entrepreneurs? Artists?

_____

_____

_____

What not-for-profit organizations are near you?

_____

_____

_____

What for-profit businesses are near you?

_____

_____

_____

What senior-citizen communities, activity centers, or nursing homes are close by?

_____

_____

_____

What government offices are near you?

_____

_____

_____

What health-food stores are in your area?

_____

_____

_____

What New Age or metaphysical bookstores are close by?

_____

_____

_____

What spas are close by?

_____

_____

_____

What clinics (free clinics, women's clinics, specialized clinics) are close?

_____

_____

_____

What hospitals are in your area?

_____

_____

_____

What artists' communities or groups of actors, musicians or writers are near you?

_____

_____

_____

What alternative or holistic healing centers are close by?

_____

_____

_____

What hair salons, sports clubs, coffee shops are nearby?

_____

_____

_____

LOCATING RESOURCES

Lists of health-food stores, spas, and practitioners can be found in the small directories you often find placed on racks or tables at the entrance to health-food stores and holistic clinics.

Hospitals can be found in the yellow pages.

Government offices, not-for-profit and for-profit organizations can be found in the white pages or by calling your local chamber of commerce and asking them to send you the most current member list or directory. It may cost you between ten and thirty-five dollars, depending on size and location, but it can be well worth the investment. Be sure to clarify how up-to-date the directory is.

Visual artists can be found in gallery directories. Go to any gallery close to you and ask how you can obtain a directory.

Actors can be found at local or regional theater companies. The chamber of commerce will have a list of the theaters in your area.

Besides finding names and addresses in directories like these, ask your friends if they can recommend any places you hadn't thought of; ask relatives and other healers. Keep expanding your list, keep adding names and phone numbers. You'll be amazed at how many prospects you can accumulate in a few weeks' time or even a few days' time. And, do understand, you're never done. Gathering these nuggets is an ongoing process for the duration of your career. My suggestion is to stay open to recommendations. You never know where they will come from.

I heard a wonderful story about this sort of serendipity from Tom LoPresti, a neuromuscular healer: Tom was sitting in LaGuardia Airport one night. His plane was delayed, as were many other flights that evening. A gentleman sat down next to him and they began a conversation — about which airline had the worse service that night, no doubt. Then one thing led to the next and they shared their occupations. It turned out that the neuromuscular healer was sitting next to a doctor who happened to be looking for a practitioner familiar with muscular tension. By the end of their delay, the doctor gave Tom his card and asked him to give him a call the next day. A few months later when I saw Tom, he couldn't wait to tell me the news. "Remember that doctor I told you about that I met at the airport? Well, I now go to his office three times a week and work with sixty percent of his patients."

WE NEVER KNOW WHEN OR HOW
THESE CONNECTIONS WILL BE MADE

This is why we need to stay open, be flexible. If we remain rigid and contracted, we'll never experience these little miracles or these random acts of kindness. We never know when we will meet someone who will enter our lives and change them in extraordinary ways. I have also come to realize that when I have been most vulnerable, and therefore most receptive, incredible life-changing events occur almost as a matter of course.

As you collect more and more names of individuals and businesses, watch what begins to happen. Your mind will start to spin with ideas. Stay with the momentum, let your imagination take off and run wild. Think about what you could offer the hospital down the street, the clinic around the corner, the health-food store in the next town, all the not-for-profit organizations who could use your services. And before any of these great ideas escape, document them on paper. Make notes regarding each one.

Do not act on any of your ideas just yet, as this is simply the "gathering nuggets" stage of your strategy, collecting all the information you can possibly find.

After you have gathered all the names and phone numbers from these various organizations, put them aside for the moment, and read through Chapter 8 — slowly and meticulously. This next chapter will help you stabilize your next steps. It will help you to deliver your message and support you in responding appropriately. So that when it is time for you to pick up the phone and call these contacts, set up appointments, you will come from a place of empowerment, rootedness, and integrity.

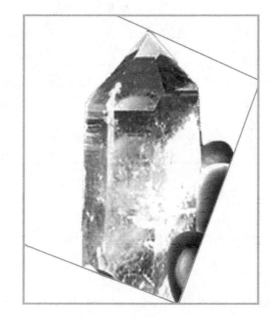

CHAPTER 8
VISUALIZING CLARITY

Visualizing Clarity

We are what we think, all that arises from our thoughts.
With our thoughts we make the world. Speak or act with a pure mind
and happiness will follow you as your unshakable shadow.

~ Buddha, the *Dhammapada*

THE PRICELESS OFFERING

Whether a client hires me for a one-time consultation or a series of coachings or decides to spend months working on a public-relations campaign, I always suggest he or she create an *offering* first. When we offer a donation or tithing to our house of faith, whether it be our church, synagogue, or spiritual community, the offering becomes a thank-you to the organization and to the very energy that supports us spiritually. When we plant flowers and grow vegetables in our gardens, we are thanking the land we live on; and our thanks comes back to us in the form of beauty and nourishment. In the same way, when we earn money through our chosen vocation, there are ways in which we can say thank you to the community in which we live. One way is by sharing our gifts.

This sharing can be a demonstration to a not-for-profit organization, an intro program to the local chamber of commerce; it can be rallying practitioners together to support the firemen at Ground Zero. The "where" doesn't matter, it's the spirit with which it is given.

There are pediatricians and heart specialists who fly to third-world countries and offer their expertise to people in need. Attorneys and successful businessmen offer their knowledge pro bono to not-for-profit organizations. Musicians raise thousands of dollars for organizations that need to promote awareness, or more research perhaps, about a disease or medical condition. These professionals do not charge for their time. They make their offering and return to their flourishing businesses. They understand on the deepest level their obligation to "give back."

I understand that the contributors I've just mentioned typically make a lot more money than most practitioners do. But, please understand, it doesn't matter how much you earn or don't earn, it's the principle of making the offering that is important.

We don't have to wait until we're successful to make this offering. In fact, the clients I've worked with who have been the most successful have made their contributions at the beginning of their careers. The results have been astounding. I just watch and see how the universe returns the favor in ways that are totally unpredictable and gratifying. Giving in this way opens us up to the universal flow of prosperity.

It is a mysterious process. Nevertheless, the more I see practitioners offering their service in this way, the more I see how it comes back in magnificent ways to those who understand this essential flow.

Cliff Shulman, the Trager practitioner and physical therapist whose bio, resumé and sound bite we've seen in Chapter 5, is a living testament to how making an offering can return to you — tenfold. Since I've known Cliff, he has been extremely busy. Besides having a thriving practice, Cliff continuously seeks out organizations that can benefit from his service. He has offered seminars and demonstrations to not-for-profit establishments such as Gilda's Club (the cancer research center established in memory of Gilda Radner) and the Arthritis Foundation. Knowing that if people like his work, they will call him back. He also understands the "anatomy of buzz," that people who appreciate his generosity will say nice things about him. Nice things spread. Cliff doesn't make the offering because of the buzz it creates, although he's smart enough to know that this is a by-product of his goodwill. He makes the offering because (1) he's a nice person and nice people do kind things; (2) he understands the law of karma, of cause and effect — that what goes around, comes around; and (3) he makes intelligent choices, so intelligent responses come back to him. Because of this understanding, these small gestures, these offerings, have returned to him in spades.

Each time Cliff offers his gift, more people inquire about his services. What's really interesting is that this wave of interest does not always come from the group he's offered his services to, but from other sources. In other words, his kindness is repaid in indirect ways.

Without fail, those who refuse to make the offering ultimately fail or remain at a stagnant place in their practice. Those who understand this concept, and make a conscious effort to perform offerings on an ongoing basis while involved in their practice, flourish. I have been a witness to this miraculous practice over and over and over. I hope you excuse my overzealous behavior when I write about this topic. It's only because I've seen it manifest impeccably so many times.

SAD BUT TRUE

I've seen the flip side manifest too. It's painful to witness, but very instructive. Cindy, a massage therapist, recently graduated from massage school. She set up shop in her condo and immediately charged high prices. She didn't increase her fees slowly while she built her practice. The day she graduated she began to charge seventy-five dollars for a massage and she didn't care who could afford her prices. Whenever she saw me, she'd whine and complain, "Please, let me know if you hear of anyone who wants a massage. I'm so desperate. Me and my husband just moved into this condo and we really need the money." All she did was gripe and complain. She never made an offering, even though I had suggested it to her on many occasions. She never had compassion for those in need. Even when a mutual friend of ours called Cindy and asked her for a massage because she was stressed out from a divorce, and had no income and two kids to feed, Cindy told our friend, "I'm sorry, but my price is seventy-five dollars. I can't reduce it, even for you. If you can't afford it, I'm sorry."

Because of this attitude and Cindy's unwillingness to be flexible under certain conditions, she is still struggling with her business and has to work two other jobs to make ends meet.

Please understand. I know your practice is a business. I fully comprehend that you have to make a living. However, there are times when you will need to put on the glasses of compassion, step outside of your head, so to speak, move into your heart — and give for the sake of giving. By remaining flexible and in your heart, you will always make the amount of money you need. It's about keeping a balance and a flow.

KEEP IT FLOWING

The first year Michael Crouch began his chiropractic practice he had lots of clients. Friends and relatives were coming to him consistently and spreading the word. And then everything seemed to stop. The flow of clients ended and his practice was at a standstill. I'd gone to see him for a treatment, because he had been highly recommended. After the session, we spoke a bit and he shared with me how surprised he was that his business had come to a complete halt. I asked him if he had made an offering lately. "Excuse me?" was his response. I explained to him what "the offering" was and could tell he really listened. I knew he understood its value. A few weeks later, I called him to see how he was doing.

He told me that an amazing thing had happened. A few days after we spoke, he'd heard that the Screen Actors Guild was putting on a health fair. "There was no money involved," he said. "But I knew it was an opportunity to make an offering. So, I took my table down to the fair and worked on hundreds of actors. Plus, I gave out gift certificates for two free visits — to bring people to my clinic." Within one month, twenty people had called him for an appointment and many of them have since become regular customers.

The last time I spoke to Michael, he told me he'd broken several records for visits — total weekly visits and total Sunday visits. He was ecstatic! He also told me that he was recently invited to attend other health fairs for not-for-profit organizations, where he'd be adjusting hundreds of cancer and arthritis patients and giving out over a thousand gift certificates.

The offering is a universal approach to creating positive buzz, applicable to every profession within any industry.

MONEY AND YOUR PRACTICE

Money, believe it not, is not the root of all evil. Money is *shakti* (energy). If more people understood this, with all its ramifications, there'd be fewer court cases, fewer divorces, no wars, more generosity, more compassion and more love.

Actors, healers, artists, musicians have long lived with the notion that poverty leads to spiritual and artistic advancement; this assumption could not be further from the truth. And yet, at some point in time, we have all become victims of this perception.

When I was studying to be an actress, I thought the more I subjected myself to struggle, the better a performer I'd become. I would put myself through the most ridiculous situations that only led to pain and suffering. I was caught up in this predicament for years and still on occasion suffer bouts of temporary insanity when I think this is the reality for a writer. No more! Trust me when I say, no more!

Haven't you seen successful writers and actors and musicians? Haven't you met successful practitioners? Don't you know in the depths of your being that you can achieve not just prosperity-consciousness, but all its joys of independence and freedom, by removing this veil of misperception?

Until we change the vibration of our thoughts and join in on the collective consciousness of financial abundance and personal power that all practitioners, healing centers, and schools desire — until we all come from a place of higher awareness, integrity, self-empowerment and professionalism — we will continue to spin on the wheel of poverty and never detach from its never-ending cycle.

There are many ways to change this cycle. For instance, today, this moment, see yourself as successful and begin to act, move, and speak from that place. Sit down every morning before you start your day and create a visualization. See yourself as abundant, as the person you see in your dreams, in your vision, and then act "as if." Not from a place of ego, but from a place of *knowing* that in your heart you are here to help people, that your service is vital to the health and well-being of many individuals, that you are a channel for divine energy to move through. And as a result of coming from that pure place of light, God-awareness, consciousness, angelic presence, *buddhi* (whatever you choose to call it), the universe will provide you with the sustenance. And this includes — yes, money.

By naming and contacting that power you call upon, embrace it, bring it into your daily visualization. Offer your work back to this source. When you move out of the place of "doership," this source can work through you and guide you to manifesting actions that will bear the best possible fruit. Continue to offer your practice, your gifts, your financial situation to this source and then move out of the way. By continually working on yourself in this way, you will attract the clientele you wish to serve.

One of the wealthiest men I know, a commodities trader on Wall Street, explained to me how to make all transactions fair. He told me this secret when I began a new business venture and asked him what I should charge clients. I wanted to be fair to my customers. I didn't want to overcharge or undercharge. He said, and I quote, "If it's fair to you and fair to the other person, it's a good deal. If it's not fair to one person, it's not a good deal."

I took his words to heart and before long discovered that the more I was sensitive to my clients' needs, the more clients were referred to me. The more I circulated money, the more money came back to me. I began to get into the flow of this circulatory state and realized that it didn't occur only when money was exchanged, it occurred when there was an *energy* exchange.

"I'll give you a neuromuscular treatment, and in exchange, you give me sixty-five dollars."

"I'll give you six Trager treatments and in exchange, will you design the first three pages of my Website?"

"I'll give you a Reiki session, if you give me fifty dollars. Oh, you can't afford fifty dollars? That's okay, I know you are also a talented hair cutter, so why don't you give me ten dollars and cut my hair? Deal?"

In other words, there's always a way to circulate money and have it work both for you and for the person you are having the exchange with.

If you can define this paradigm for yourself and truly understand that money is about giving and receiving and that there's a billion ways for this energy to be exchanged, you'll never have to feel guilty about discussing money with clients or asking for money or receiving money again. Think of all the possibilities that would open up for you when talking to patients who perhaps can't afford your services. It's beyond barter. It's energy in exchange for energy.

Lakshmi, the goddess of wealth in the Hindu tradition, is most often portrayed sitting upon a full-blown lotus. Lakshmi brings growth, generosity, and abundance to whatever is life-enhancing. We often see her with one or two of her hands fully open, radiating showers of gold coins. Or when one hand alone is pouring coins, the other is often depicted with an open palm facing outward, poised in the gesture of blessing that means "fear not." The fact that these coins are flowing in a constant stream indicates that this is an active, ongoing, conscious process. This gesture might also serve as an inherent reminder that the stream can indeed be stopped, should our invocation and honoring of her gifts cease to flow from us with sincerity and devotion.

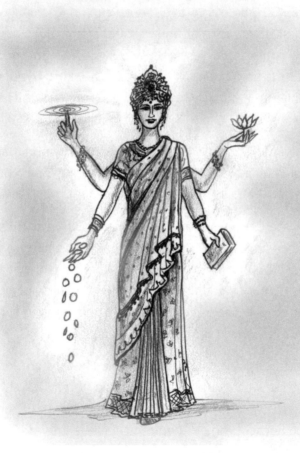

How can I keep Lakshmi flowing in my life and in my practice?

Here's an interesting story that might help plant this message more firmly in your heart:

There was a successful orthodontist in Northampton, Massachusetts. I'll refer to her as Dr. Rutherford for the sake of confidentiality. Rumor had it that Dr. Rutherford was by far the best orthodontist in all of New England. She had three offices throughout the state and there were children on waiting lists at all three. I was a single parent, starting my own business, and could not afford braces for my son, although he needed them badly. So I set up an appointment to meet Dr. Rutherford (I figured I might as well start with the best). I explained my situation and asked if she would consider a barter since I was starting my own PR firm. Without pausing, she invited me to lunch. I couldn't believe it. We met at a lovely restaurant the following week and she explained how she'd been thinking of ways to create a more family environment with all three offices — somehow tie them all together. I suggested creating a newsletter that would involve all her patients, all the children she served. They could submit articles and jokes and poems, draw pictures of themselves before and after the braces. We could have a contest to name the newsletter. She loved the idea and we shook hands. It was a great deal.

I created the newsletter *Brace Yourself* for three years on a bimonthly basis and Dr. Rutherford took care of all my son's orthodontic needs. It was a fabulous exchange. It became no surprise to me why her practice was so successful. I must have told fifty people about her generosity and several of my friends ended up going to her. And who knows how many other people heard about how great she was?

CREATIVE WAYS TO CHARGE

Because most health-insurance plans do not cover his services, Evan Fleischmann, ND, believes that money should never be a barrier to proper health care. Therefore he offers his services on a sliding-scale basis. Dr. Fleischmann's first comprehensive visit takes about two hours, and for that he gives his patients the option of paying between one hundred and three hundred dollars. Whatever they feel comfortable paying. Follow-up visits take approximately 45 minutes to an hour, and for that he asks between fifty and one hundred and fifty dollars. Any supplements that may be indicated are additional, and he discounts them for his patients as well.

Joe Miglierie is a chiropractor from Northfield, New Jersey. Joe's practice, Peak Performance, uses what is called the "honor fee system" or "the box on the wall." This concept has been in existence for over thirty years and was used exclusively when chiropractic work was a "cash only" business and, in some places, illegal. Joe adopted this payment system because he feels it is the purest form of payment and one way an entire family can come for spinal checkups on a regular basis, no matter what they can afford.

The reason Joe uses the honor fee system is because, like Dr. Fleischmann, Joe has a strong belief that no price can be placed on health. "Chiropractic care," he says, "should be made available to every human being, so they can express Life to their maximum potential."

The way the honor fee system works is: each person pays according to his or her ability. If Joe were to charge a set amount there would always be someone who could not afford that fee. And since every person knows his or her own financial status, Joe created a system that allows every patient to set a flat weekly fee that is honest, reasonable, and within each person's financial means.

This system is not designed to be a charity or a bargain, nor is it to be taken advantage of. Joe explains that it is a privilege, and an obligation, to offer in this way.

The three obligations that must be met in order for patients to participate in this fee system are:

1. Be regular with your visits (a minimum of once a week).
2. Pay the weekly fee that you have set on the first visit of each week.
3. Refer others to this office.

If a patient's financial situation changes it is the patient's responsibility to adjust the fee accordingly. All Joe asks is that the patient tell him that his or her situation has changed. A change for the worse in a financial situation is not a reason to miss your weekly spinal checkup.

Now here is a perfect example of thinking "outside the box" by going "inside the box."

IT ALL COMES DOWN TO SELF-WORTH

If Joe didn't feel worthy of receiving a just amount from his clients, he would starve. If he didn't have the attitude of gratitude, he would not attract people who were thankful for his unique billing system. What thoughts are you thinking and putting out there about worthiness?

Another Joe, Joe Lubow, executive director of the Sarasota School of Massage Therapy, told me an interesting story. He said he knew a therapist who charged a hundred and twenty dollars for a ten-minute session. Someone asked the therapist how he had the nerve to charge such an enormous amount of money for so little time. The therapist said, "I charge ten dollars for what I *do* and a hundred and ten dollars for what I *know*."

On the other hand, there are practitioners who determine a set price for their patients and stay firm. They do not barter and have made the decision to offer charity through other means. Find what works for you, find the balance in your giving and in your receiving. When the flow stops, stop and reevaluate your situation. Take a look at your priorities, see where they might have changed, and then make the necessary and appropriate transition.

THE POWER OF THE WORD

Death and Life are in the power of the tongue.

~ Proverbs 18:21

How many times have you been absolutely elated when someone called you on the phone and told you how much they appreciated having you in their life? How many times have you felt irritated because someone was rude to you on the subway or at work, using words that attacked you? We are all affected by what other people say to us. Rare is the person who can allow words to scatter off them like pellets of water and not be affected by praise or blame. The truth of the matter is, until we've reached that state of detachment — even better, enlightenment — it is critical that we stay conscious of the words we choose while communicating with others.

There is a term in the Sanskrit language that describes this concept precisely: *matrika shakti*. It's also my favorite expression, as it epitomizes the importance of how one word can have so much power. *Matrika shakti* literally means the energy of the word — the charge of the word. In the *Shiva Sutras,* a highly respected treatise from the ancient Indian philosophy of Kashmir Shaivism, it is explained how sound itself carries thought and intention, and thus creates a vibratory response, not only in the person saying the word, but in the vibration that goes out into the air, which is absorbed by another person, and by the creation itself.

WORDS CARRY VIBRATIONS

So if we could imagine that every word we speak has this vibratory power and that this reverberation gets carried out into the universe whenever we voice a word out loud, we would get a glimpse of how important it is to be careful of every word we say. Not only that, but each vibratory response corre- 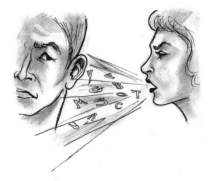 sponds with a specific feeling. It can be a feeling of happiness, a feeling of embarrassment, humiliation, depression. Every one of these emotions affects our subtle system, and becomes a part of our physical being.

Even when we say words silently to ourselves — like "You are such an idiot, how could you have forgotten that appointment?" or "I'm so proud of you for treating the patient the way you did" — these silent mantras we repeat to ourselves, which no one else hears, also carry a corresponding emotion. And each emotion gets recorded in our soul. Every one gets lodged in our subtle body. I've heard this a number of times from Carolyn Myss, a medical intuitive and the author of many books, including *Anatomy of the Spirit:* "Every feeling we experience," she says, "leaves a deep impression." Words with negative connotations leave negative impressions. Words with positive connotations leave positive impressions. Positive or negative, they both take up residence in our bodies, and eventually, those negative impressions reveal themselves and we reexperience them — through illness. Wherever we are at our weakest, our bodies will manifest those masked emotions.

Gurumayi Chidvilasananda, the Siddha Yoga meditation master, has said, "We are born into a state of bliss. The only reason we change from that state is due to matrika shakti."

So wouldn't you say we all have a responsibility to make sure the words we are saying — even thinking — are uplifting?

Especially practitioners, as it's your presence as much as your skill that is the precious vehicle through which others seek healing. You are the safety net, the cushion for these clients to feel secure with, as they come to be soothed, stroked and embraced. They come to you because they've been beaten, or they've lost their jobs or they've been in accidents or they're simply stressed out. They are vulnerable and feel exposed and need to trust someone with their open wounds. Can they trust you?

WHEN ANGER IS BEHIND YOUR WORDS, ANGER IS WHAT PEOPLE WILL FEEL

Several years ago, Amy, a friend of mine, called a massage therapist she'd heard positive things about and set up an appointment to meet her. Amy was feeling very overwhelmed; her son was mentally ill, her husband was talking about a divorce. This was not a happy time for

Amy. She really needed to be in a peaceful environment, even for an hour. The massage therapist began to work on her and was a few minutes into the session when the phone rang. The therapist left Amy on the table, picked up the phone and began to mouth obscenities to her boyfriend. "Get your goddam clothes out of my house before I get home or I'm calling the police" . . . pause . . . "I don't give a f— why you can't get there before . . ." pause . . .

It was more than Amy could deal with. When the therapist returned to my friend, Amy had already begun to put her clothes back on and was about to leave. The therapist apologized for the intrusion and said, "Look, I'll give you a discount for the massage." Amy thanked the therapist and explained to her that it was too much for her right now. Well, the massage therapist had a hissy fit and started yelling. "Let's just finish up here, all right? I'll turn off the phone."

Amy told me she didn't know what to say. All she knew was that she had to leave, that she couldn't handle the energy the therapist was putting out even if she'd offered her a discount.

And even beyond the words, what's going on *behind* them? Even if you say the nicest thing to someone, if there is anger behind what you say, anger is what they will walk away and vibrate with.

There was a study done at the University of Michigan's communication department several years ago. The department created a survey to determine what people were affected by most: body language, word content, or voice tone. Any ideas as to what their findings showed? People were most affected by voice tone. Body language was second and word content was last.

Be aware of your words and the thoughts behind your words. Check your state. Of course, we're not saints yet, and it's a challenge to be in a constant state of bliss — all the time. Boy, I sure try! But if you're aware that you're not in a good space, you may want to take precautionary measures not to let any of the negativity affect your work. Meditate, chant, pray, sit in front of a candle, do whatever it is you do to disarm these *vrittis* (another Sanskrit term meaning the manifestations or waves of the mind) lest they take charge. Be aware of the thoughts behind your words, as their subtle vibrations can ultimately make or break your practice, and your very effectiveness as a healer.

THE SUBTEXT OF ENTHUSIASM

In the same way that a Reiki practitioner will not administer Reiki without a prayer, without a particular subtext embodied through his or her touch, a person making a telephone call or meeting someone for the first time also needs to have a subtext. Allow me to suggest one: enthusiasm.

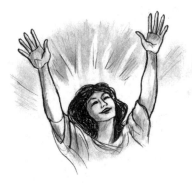

Enthusiasm is more powerful than salesmanship, stronger than the gift of gab, more profound than good looks. In fact, I can't think of anything that reveals one's state of mind, one's character, one's integrity and one's love for what one does more than enthusiasm. Look at Oprah, Jeff Bezos of Amazon.com, Suze Orman, author of *The Courage to Be Rich,* or Tony Robbins, the great motivational speaker. Each of them displays a tremendous enthusiasm when they talk about what they do. People can't help but listen to them and be affected by their state.

As enthusiastic as these individuals are, not all of us have this kind of personality, nor is it always appropriate to act out this kind of exuberance in our practice. Enthusiasm is not always about jumping up and down and grinning from ear to ear. Enthusiasm can be subtle and it can manifest by the simple bubbling up of your concern, love and compassion for the person you're talking to, be it on the phone or in person.

Your positive energy will create a more lasting effect on others than the most eloquent, well-spoken sound bite in the world. So, when it comes time for you to go out there and meet people or pick up the phone to set up an appointment, remember to place the subtext of enthusiasm behind your words.

In addition:
- Be articulate.
- Be sincere.
- Be humble.
- Be discriminating.

COMPETITION ~ AND THE FACT THAT THERE IS NONE

What seems different in yourself: that's the rare thing you possess.
The one thing that gives each of us his worth, and that's just what we try
to suppress. And we claim to "love thyself"?
~ Andre Gide

"*The mood of competition is a sure recipe for failure.* It is a stance that is in a chronic stage of vigilance, a body that stiffens and pushes against a perceived opponent," Richard Strozzi Heckler declares in his book *Holding the Center.*

Don't you feel what it's like when you are in that state? There is no giving or sharing of information, of gifts, of contacts, of anything.

Competition is nothing more than a state of contraction. It never stimulates healthy interactions, expansion, or creativity; it only brings about stiffness and distance.

We have the tendency to compete:

- when we listen to others and feel "less than";
- when we are jealous of someone else's good fortune;
- when we want to uplift ourselves from a negative state of mind.

The addiction of competition will subside when we stop looking at others and respond only to our own truth.

Know that if there are twenty acupuncturists in the same city, residing on the same block, there is still no need for the stance of competition.

Each one of these acupuncturists is unique, with his or her own set of values, his or her own way of administering experientially gleaned knowledge, and his or her own energy that will resonate with some clients and not necessarily with others.

When the mood of competition arises, we need only to ask ourselves:

Am I doing what I love?

_____

_____

Is there a choice for me to be doing something different?

_____

_____

_____

What makes me unique?

_____

_____

_____

_____

_____

Think about those individuals who are in professions similar to yours. Who are they?

_____

_____

_____

_____

_____

_____

_____

_____

_____

_____

_____

_____

What is it they do that you think is great and is working for them?

_____

_____

_____

_____

_____

_____

_____

_____

Is there anything they do that you feel is unacceptable?

_____

_____

_____

_____

_____

_____

_____

If they are successful, why are they?

_____

_____

_____

_____

_____

_____

_____

_____

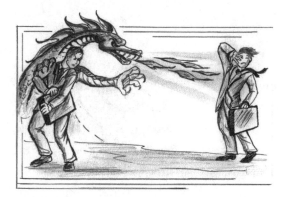

When we see the dragon's head of envy rise up, wanting to bite off the legs of others to make ourselves look taller; when we experience inadequacies in ourselves or when we feel "less than": stop! Check inside and ask if it is necessary to proceed with this present form of action or if there is a choice for you to travel a higher road.

YOUR PRACTICE IS GREATER
THAN YOU BELIEVE IT TO BE

I read an amazing book some years ago on the topic of fundraising. I'm embarrassed to admit that I have since forgotten the name of this book, especially when it made such a huge impact on my work. Nevertheless, the essence of its message was a demonstration that successful fundraising comes from convincing donors that the purpose for which funds are being raised, and the impact of a donor's gifting, are more significant than the potential donor believes them to be.

Let me explain. When I was raising money for the Council on Alcoholism and Drug Abuse, most donors thought I was raising money only to fix up the alcohol and drug treatment facility, because it was on its last legs. Well, that was partly true; the council did need money for building expenses quite badly. But it was just as important for donors to understand that part of their donation would go toward the various programs the council offered, like the Kids Klub, a creative after-school program for children whose parents were either in jail or on probation because of drugs or alcohol. There was a camp initiative, to provide an opportunity for these kids to leave their dysfunctional homes for a week and experience healthy activities and friendships, see that there was a better life they deserved and could strive for. I gave donors a list of all the programs their gifts could be earmarked for. They had no idea the council had so many initiatives. They appreciated the fact that I was informing them. The council became much greater to them than they'd thought it was and this new vision made all the difference in my ability to raise hundreds of thousands of dollars.

When you understand your service is greater than what you believe it to be — when you see your practice from a broader perspective, rather than an individual one — then it becomes easier for you to offer your services, it becomes easier for you to educate clients, potential hosts and partners.

Here's the thought process.

If I were talking to the director of human resources or to the president of a company to explain to him the benefits of teaching the Alexander technique to his employees, this is what I'd say:

This technique not only helps people to sit straight and have better posture. After a very short time, your staff will feel so much better about themselves and about the work environment that, most likely, productivity will increase, relationships will improve, people's sense of well-being will be enhanced. Your employees may even enjoy coming to work so much, they may want to stay later and come in earlier.

By expanding your profession beyond the conventional form as you know it, you will help others understand its profound significance for themselves and for the world around them. Everything has its ripple effect. You're simply describing how your practice creates its own ripple.

SELLING **AS A DIVINE PRACTICE**

Life's most urgent question is, what are you doing for others?
~ Martin Luther King, Jr.

I purposely made the word *selling* small, so as not to turn some of you off before you have a chance to read what I have to say about the subject.

The word *selling* has had such a bad connotation for so many years that no matter where people go with their thoughts concerning the word, it's usually in a discouraging direction. For me as for most people, negative thoughts used to bubble up in my mind whenever I thought of the word. To discover the truth of this for yourself, try this experiment: inside the circle below, write the word *selling*.

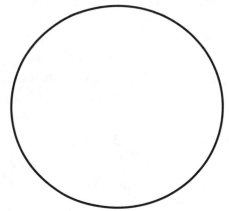

Now, around the word *selling*, write every word that comes to mind when you think of the word.

When I have received these diagrams back from people in my workshops, I've usually seen words like *manipulation, coercion, pushy, conniving, peddling, underhanded, power tripping, dishonest, crass.*

The question to ask ourselves is not only what words come to mind when we contemplate this action. The question to ask is, are we guilty of creating any of these feelings in other people when we approach them about our practice? Are we being manipulative, or pushy, or demonstrating coercion? Are we selling people something they don't want or need? If we have the slightest sense that we are, then we are.

When we act in a falsely demonstrative way, it's usually because we're insecure — about money, position, competition or success. Or perhaps it's an old habit from childhood, when we found that the only way we could get that toy car we saw in the window or that cool new red bicycle was by being manipulative or flirtatious. As we grew older and more sophisticated, we wanted bigger and better toys; we wanted people to change their minds to "our side." We wanted people to hire us, be our friend, love us. Unconsciously, we became quite adept at being coercive and cunning.

How many times have you tried talking a friend into doing something you knew in advance they didn't want to do? Even if it was something as innocent as going to the movies? I have a friend who used to do this to me constantly. Finally, I mentioned something to him about this habit and he stopped, but until I did, it had almost ruined a wonderful relationship. If we are creating this behavior unconsciously, to try to get clients, we need to look inside and figure out what is provoking the behavior.

People sense our needs, our insecurities, even if they don't verbalize it. They sense our energy, the vibe we're "putting out there." What vibe do you want out there, representing you? A needy vibe? A powerful "I can help you" vibe? A begging "Please, come to see me" vibe? "I can heal you" (trust me) vibe? Really take a close look at how you are handling this subtle approach to people when you meet them.

> *When we come*
> *from the place of love, from service,*
> *people will never have the impression*
> *that we are selling them a bill of goods*
> *they don't want.*

A FORCE OF NATURE

My entire concept of selling was transformed after spending a few evenings with Patricia Bragg, the health crusader whose portrait is on every bottle of Braggs Liquid Aminos, Braggs Organic Apple Cider Vinegar, Braggs Organic Olive Oil and array of other healthful Bragg products. After I was introduced to Patricia, my understanding of the word *selling* changed forever.

Upon my first meeting with this dynamic force of nature, I was enraptured by her vibrant vitality. Her petite frame was in counterpoint to her huge smile that lit up her entire garden, and when she looked at you, you knew you were the only person who existed in her universe. Within minutes of shaking my hand and introducing herself to me, she handed me a bag filled with Bragg products and said to me, "It's a gift. Please take them. Use them for yourself or pass them out to your friends." Then she whisked me off to the movies, to see *Ya Ya Sisterhood*. An appropriate film, since I felt like we'd been sisters for at least two or three past lives.

When we stepped out of the car to enter the theater, she had yet another bag filled with brochures and books that she proceeded to pass out to strangers, as well as to people who had recognized her.

She'd hand them each a book and whisper in their ear, "This will be very healthy information for you, please read it," then she'd be off sailing through the crowd like a schoolgirl with her notoriuos petaled Easter bonnet (her insignia on all her products), handing yet another book to yet another passerby. She must have passed out at least fifteen books between the parking lot and the entrance to the movie theater. Everyone smiled and seemed pleased to receive her gift.

As soon as the movie was over, more books and brochures were pulled from her bag and given to people in the lobby, standing in line for the next show. At first I thought maybe she was just putting on this show to impress me (the new girl in town) or maybe she just did this at the movies. But when we pulled into the local diner to get a bite to eat, and sat down at the counter, not two seconds went by before she popped up and started walking around the main dining area handing out books and brochures to patrons while they ate.

Now, Patricia is a woman who doesn't have to sell anything. Her products are known and used throughout the world. She could easily sit back and reap the benefits from her good fortune. But Patricia

Bragg is clearly on a mission and it goes far beyond any thought of establishing her name and fame or needing to get her products to a larger audience. She is the consummate health crusader, eager to educate people about health options. I couldn't believe my good fortune, being in this woman's presence, watching this sweet strawberry blonde take on the neighborhood. What amazing lessons this taught me.

- Don't play small.
- Don't keep your gifts a secret.
- Share the love.

When we put into practice these three jewels with the other points offered in this chapter, the old negative concept of selling will not enter our consciousness. The word *selling* itself will no longer affect us in the same way. Our entire *modus operandi* will change. In fact, we'll begin to experience this *gift of giving,* in this new way, and may even begin to *love to SELL.* Because we're coming from a pure place when we do it.

You can get everything
you want in life --
if you help enough people
get what they want.

~ Zig Zeigler, *See You at the Top*

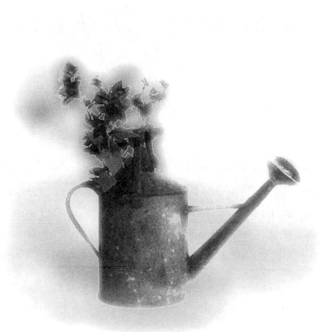

CHAPTER 9

WATERING THE SEEDS OF ABUNDANCE

Watering the Seeds of Abundance

It is right in your face.
This moment the whole thing is handed to you.

~ *Tao te Ching*

You've completed your gathering. You have all your lists. You have your resumé, your bio, your sound bite. You have the right understanding about the words you are going to use, and you have your subtext of enthusiasm. Think about who you would like to call first from your list. It's time to water the seeds that you've planted.

Before you make any of those calls, however, you may want to create a *contact sheet*. It will make life ten times easier and more organized.

THE CONTACT SHEET

The contact sheet is a practical tool you can use while making telephone calls to individuals and organizations. Every time you make a call, you can use this designated format (see next page) to write down the date, the organization you've telephoned, the phone number, the name of the person you've spoken to, their response, and when you should call them back. This way you'll have everything you need in one glance, on one sheet.

In one glance, you'll know that you called the Arthritis Foundation on May 26; the person you spoke to was Maryanne

Jacoby. She was very interested in what you had to say but asked that you please call her back. You have her phone number and her extension and the date she asked you to call her back on.

You can make up separate contact sheets for each type of outreach you are doing. For instance, you can have contact sheets for workshops, offerings, and potential sponsors. The best thing about this piece of paper is that everything is organized in one place and can be a terrific reference for you during the weeks and months ahead. When you create your own contact sheet, you may want to use the categories listed below, placed horizontally on the page, as seen here:

Date   Company   Contact   Phone   E-mail   Website   Response   Call back

WHILE ON THE PHONE, THINK ABOUT A STRATEGIC ALLIANCE

Not too long ago, a merger took place I'm sure you heard about. One of the largest Internet service providers, AOL, and the most prestigious television network, TimeWarner, became partners in one of the biggest alliances in U.S. history. Why did these two companies decide to partner? What motivated them to join forces? I can only guess at a few of the reasons:

1. They knew they could make a more profound impact on consumers' lives.

2. They knew that with collaboration, they could improve not only the way people communicated, but the way viewers are entertained.

3. The coming together of their instruments, the TV and the computer, would give these companies the opportunity to pursue their goals in a powerful new way that would ultimately change the way every single person watches and interacts with his or her television set.

4. They knew they could never achieve this dream by remaining autonomous.

Perhaps this is an elaborate example of creating a strategic alliance. But I wanted to demonstrate that if this kind of relationship can work with two gigantic corporations — with all their intricate infrastructure and all their glorified egos — why can't it happen with practitioners and healing institutions?

Some of you may think these two companies were simply acting out of greed, the need to monopolize the industry, the intent to stomp on smaller companies trying to get ahead in the same game. And perhaps that is partly true. I happen to think these two companies have taken advantage of their extraordinary vision and the timeliness of where the next generation of TV watchers and computer users ultimately want to be, and whether we like it or not will produce an interactive TV, the likes of which we have never imagined.

Many of you practitioners may have no interest in the computer or in watching television, and so this example, in your eyes, may seem to be an odd choice. Nevertheless, there is something to be learned from these two megastructures that have joined forces, and that is: whether it is a permanent merger or a limited partnership, the right partnering can add strength to any practice, to any organization, and serve more people more effectively.

When it comes to partnering, many practitioners and healing centers have shown a lot of fear: fear of expansion, a desire to remain in isolation, to maintain a certain elitism. When we blind ourselves to the potentiality of what can be gained by coming together and sharing assets and ideas, we lose sight of our obligation to serve a larger community — and by doing so have missed an essential window to grow beyond our limited universe.

As long as we allow such a narrow way of thinking to persist, we block the process of the collective mind's maturing and the possibility of waking up to experiencing the garden of prosperity.

AN IDEAL PARTNERSHIP

An example of a wonderful partnership arose when a holistic retreat center asked me to develop a marketing plan for their organization. I wanted to provide them with a plan that would benefit their retreat center, the practitioner population they served, and the neighboring corporations surrounding them. Tapping into the natural synergy between these three sets of interests, we came up with a plan that would serve them all equally.

It is common knowledge that employees experience stress in the workplace. Just sitting at the computer all day, workers can develop backaches and neck aches, carpal tunnel syndrome, bad vision, bad attitudes and lack of energy, to name only a few of the chronic "dis-eases" they endure.

Located only miles away from a cluster of corporations, the retreat center held many of the solutions to the everyday problems these corporations and their employees faced. The retreat center staff and I knew that their practitioners held a key to prevention of the repetition of these chronic ailments. All we had to do was to introduce their services to the corporations.

Through the comprehensive program we developed, the professionally trained practitioners affiliated with the retreat center presented to the corporations a menu of therapies: relaxation, Alexander Technique, acupressure, Reiki, shiatsu, hypnotherapy. For an annual fee, corporations would pay the retreat center for selected services from the menu for their employees. The benefits of this relationship were threefold:

- Employees would experience more energy, increased creativity, better communication, and a healthier work environment.

- Corporations in turn would benefit by the reduction of sick time, enhanced employee productivity and decision making, overall improved morale and wellness, and better vibes among the employees and management.

- And finally, the retreat center would then provide more work for their holistic healers, with increased revenue to run a more efficient organization.

Everybody wins! Everybody did win. Top management from several of the corporations began to request more massage therapists. They began to reward their employees with a massage every time employee achievements went beyond the norm. Soon employees were working harder. There was more team effort, business increased. More body-workers were employed, and the retreat center's good reputation spread throughout the region.

NOT-FOR-PROFIT SPONSORS

If you are thinking about creating a seminar, a workshop or any kind of presentation, you may want to think about finding an organization to sponsor or host it for you. If it's the right match, the organization will have as much to gain from this collaboration as you will. The first thing you'll want to do is contemplate the kind of organization you want to be affiliated with. Think of it as if you were expanding your own team for a short time. What kind of team members would you select? What would be the qualities you'd look for? What kind of collaboration would you need?

A former client of mine, Joanne Ehret, an acupuncturist and Chinese herbal medicine practitioner whose resumé and bio we've seen in Chapter 4, was seeking to reach a higher echelon of clientele. I suggested we hold a program at Smith College in Northampton, Massachusetts. It was a prime venue: there were five universities within a five-mile radius, one of them huge, the others extremely prestigious.

The timing was perfect. Springtime was approaching and allergy sufferers wanted alternatives to allopathic medications. My client grasped the power of the moment and called the presentation "Chinese Medicine and Springtime Maladies: Exploring a traditional paradigm of healing to reframe and redefine asthma and allergies" — which satisfied the listeners' ears and the colleges' love for long titles.

I arranged for the anthropology department to sponsor the event, which otherwise would have cost my client hundreds of dollars in insurance and rental fees. The event was a huge success, as each party met their goals: Joanne educated her community about the benefits of Chinese herbs and acupuncture. The university created an outreach program that bridged the gap between their institution and the greater community. The audience was able to receive answers to questions regarding acupuncture and Chinese herbs, and some practical new approaches to their own health concerns.

This alliance brought Joanne the academic clientele she'd desired, and the university was praised for creating a successful community event.

Who doesn't want their name affiliated with something good? What organization doesn't want their name spread around town as a forward-looking presenter of an informative event? All you have to do is point out the reasons why it is to a potential host organization's benefit to sponsor you, and look for organizations who will:

- add substance to your presentation,
- have an interest in what you do,
- support you in the outreach,
- share their resources,
- bring energy and enthusiasm,
- and share in the risk and in the rewards.

Here are a few more reasons why selecting a not-for-profit organization to team up with is advantageous:

1. You rarely, if ever, have to pay for advertising. And if you do, the media will offer you a lower rate, as they have not-for-profit rates.

2. Such an organization usually has a significant membership base and a formidable mailing list.

3. Reporters will be more apt to write about your event.

4. You can receive discounts on printing costs and mailings through your partner's not-for-profit 501(c)3 status.

5. By offering the not-for-profit's members a percentage of your event (if you charge), you automatically create that anatomy of buzz, for they too have benefitted by your presence. And believe me, the buzz that is generated from this act of goodwill lasts much longer than the event. Your name lives on and your admirable reputation travels.

THE AGREEMENT

Regardless of the kind of relationship you have committed to with another organization, be it a partnering situation for one event or a cluster of workshops that you will be teaming up to present, a contract should be written to specify what the responsibilities are for each of you for the time you will be working together. This agreement does not have to be elaborate. Its purpose is to achieve clarity by stating what your sponsor or partner has agreed to do and what you have agreed to do.

For instance, the sponsor or partner may agree to:

- provide the space;
- advertise in their local newspaper or magazine;
- send out a press release;
- distribute flyers to their membership;
- send out invitations to their members;
- pay for advertisements in local newspapers.

You may agree to:

- write the press release;
- write the flyer;
- distribute flyers to the community;
- send invitations to targeted audience.

The sponsoring organization may ask you to compose and print up all the promotional materials, with the arrangement to reimburse you at the end of the event. If this responsibility falls to you, make sure you get it in writing (see sample agreement on the next page) and save all your receipts. With everything written down in black and white, there will be no surprises or misunderstandings at the end of the day. Everyone will see clearly what each party is responsible for.

AGREEMENT BETWEEN JANICE DOE
and the HOLISTIC CENTER OF WASHINGTON

This is an agreement between JANICE DOE of 38390 Greystone Place, Suite K, Riverdale, NY 10463, and the sponsoring organization, THE HOLISTIC CENTER OF WASHINGTON, Studio 9, Washington, DC 87409. JANICE DOE agrees to present the workshop "What Is Acupuncture" on MAY 18, 2002, to be held at _____, located at_____.

The workshop will begin at 1:00 and will end at approximatly 5:00 pm on the same day.

The cost of the workshop will be $125.00 per person.

THE HOLISTIC CENTER OF WASHINGTON shall receive 15% of the net proceeds from the workshop AND shall receive ONE FREE ADMISSION for the course, if there are 20 participants or more. If the number of participants drops below 20, the percentage will be 10%.

JANICE DOE will provide brochures and a fully formatted flyer that can be used for advertising and will provide all text needed to promote the event.

JANICE DOE agrees to:
1. Provide sponsor with all marketing materials, including: a fully formatted flyer that can be used for advertising; a press release.
2. Make all travel arrangements and lay out initial payment for all travel and food. Travel and food will be reimbursed to JANICE DOE after the conclusion of the workshop, and the amount therefor shall be deducted

from the gross proceeds before percentages are computed for The Holistic Center of Washington and JANICE DOE, respectively.

THE HOLISTIC CENTER OF WASHINGTON agrees to:

1. Provide the space for the workshop at no additional cost to JANICE DOE;
2. Advertise in local newspapers;
3. Promote the workshop in its newsletter;
4. Distribute flyers to members and other appropriate establishments;
5. Register participants and keep JANICE DOE informed and up-to-date with the numbers of participants so registered;
6. Collect checks, money orders and cash from participants for the course; deposit all monies and write a check to JANICE DOE for (a) travel/food expenses plus (b) 85% to 90% of the net, as specified above, at the end of the course in U.S. currency.

SIGNATORIES:

JANICE DOE, Licensed Acupuncturist

_____

THE HOLISTIC CENTER OF WASHINGTON

_____

By: John Smith, DC, Executive Director

DATE: _____

INTERNET POSSIBILITIES

In the Winter 2001 issue of *Massage Therapy* magazine, there was an entire segment dedicated to the "Hottest Massage and Holistic Practitioner Websites." I was amazed at how many sites there were representing this population and how fast it was growing, how many practitioners were being certified and at what pace.

It is no longer astonishing to see how the communication age has affected the complementary-health industry. For years, practitioners didn't want to go near a computer, for many reasons: EMFs, bad karma, energetically it didn't feel right. Even today, there are practitioners who want nothing to do with a computer.

Many of you will want to remain local and not want to venture out further than your immediate area, as you are doing quite well serving local people. However, for those healers offering their service long distance, via the telephone, e-mail, CDs, cassettes, and chats, there are virtually (no pun intended) millions of ways to connect with people who may need your services — through cyberspace.

One of the ways you can communicate with your client base and beyond is by creating an e-mail newsletter. This is a great way to market your service and at the same time keep the loyalty of your clients. Besides, there are no printing costs, no mailing costs. It's less time-consuming than a hard-copy newsletter and faster than any mail you could possibly send.

By generating an e-mail newsletter, you have free rein to write about an array of topics that will be of interest to your clients. You can write about recent research, announce new workshops, courses, or discounts. Interview people introducing new modalities. Have a question-and-answer column.

Start conservatively. Send the newsletter out once, then repeat every two months at first. Then, when you see that people are interested and you hear positive responses, send one every month. Start slow and pace yourself. You may find that the newsletter takes off and that you may even need to hire someone to help you. (More about e-mail newsletters in Chapter 11.)

This virtual marketing technique will:
- remind your clients that you care,
- create goodwill,
- give them another reason to come see you.

E-MAIL SIGNATURE

An e-mail signature allows you to add your contact information at the bottom of every e-mail you send. This way, in case you forget to mention that you have a Website, for instance, every communication will automatically display the Website address, your phone number, your fax number and your e-mail address as part of your signature.

This is the e-mail signature I am currently using:

Andrea Adler,
Author of PR FOR THE HOLISTIC HEALER
  and CREATING AN ABUNDANT PRACTICE;
Workshop presenter, speaker, consultant/coach,
www.HolisticPR.com

Here are a few signature etiquette rules to follow:

- Keep it short, four to six lines at most. You will see longer sigs, but for the most part they are a turn-off.
- Try not to have your sig longer than your e-mail.
- Avoid whole sentences. Do not use exclamation points.

Check with your Internet provider or e-mail program to see how to create your signature.

WEBSITES

Only a few years ago, it might have cost thousands of dollars to create a Website. Now, there are classes in everything from basic Web design to sophisticated graphics, including how to use HTML so you can edit your own site. These courses have made it easy for many people to learn how to create and manage their own sites. However, if you are not one of those do-it-your-selfers, and have no time or patience to create your own Website, you can call a consultant. They can help steer you in the right direction, and if you get stuck, they're close by to "unstick" you. There should be several listed in the yellow pages or in your local newspaper.

Perhaps you're on a limited budget. If that's the case, one idea might be to telephone one of the high schools or community colleges in your area and ask to speak to the head of the computer department. Ask them if they would recommend a qualified student who might help you create a Website. A lot of these talented teens are whizzes at the computer and they charge a lot less than a professional consultant. Like interns, these students can be very responsible, very eager to make a little money and place this work experience on their resumé.

Having a Website these days is as common as having a brochure. The Website is the new calling card. Only a Website allows millions of viewers to see who you are in a very convenient, expeditious way. By having one, the message you transmit to people is that you are serious about your work and you are here for the long haul. If you already have a brochure, you can pretty much include the brochure text on your Website or build your site around it as a framework.

In the same way that you assessed others' graphics to create your brochure, search the Internet for sites you like and then incorporate their qualities into your own Website. Remember, you don't have to build twenty pages when you first start your site; you can begin with one or two pages and add pages when you have more time and more information.

Basically, you want to welcome visitors from all walks of life to your site and let them know who you are, what your service is about, the population you serve, and how they can get in touch with you. You will want your pages to be inviting and beautiful to look at, easy on the eyes. Some sites that at first glance seem colorful and animated, using flash and shockwave applications, create stress on the eyes. A lot of people do not find it comforting to stay on this kind of site for very long. The longer someone stays on your site, the better the job you've accomplished in creating your design.

LINK TO OTHER SITES

Once your site is up and running, make sure you include a link whereby people can e-mail you directly. This way, if visitors have questions, they have a way of contacting you immediately — and the energy and impetus of their discovering you goes right into action.

Another way to market your practice or healing center is to link with other complementary providers. Link with health-food stores, other practitioners, wholesalers, distributors. Think outside of the box and write down all the places that might be interested in co-branding your e-mail newsletter, for instance. You'll have access to barter opportunities you never dreamed might be possible.

Surf the Web, see what sites you might want to link with. Everyone wants exposure. Linking with other sites is a great way to generate that exposure and, at the same time, share the wealth. More traffic will move from one site to another — energetically your name will move through the World Wide Web from one continent to another — and both your sites will get recognized faster.

By linking with other sites, you'll be able to:
- offer your books to a larger audience;
- provide more people with the schedule of your workshops;
- have thousands of people view or buy your e-mail newsletter.

Who knows, in the not-so-distant future you may want to present a *live* chat, using streaming media to capture you in action — *showing* people what you do in addition to *telling* people what you do.

Once you set your cyber-intentions in motion, there is no end to the infinite possibilities that can manifest.

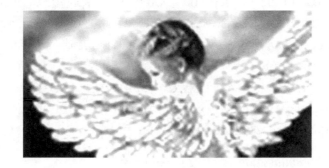

CHAPTER 10

SPREADING YOUR WINGS

Spreading Your Wings

The movement of heaven is full of power.
It furthers one to install helpers and to set armies marching.

~ the *I Ching*

This is the part of the journey where you begin to spread your wings and expand on all levels. This is where you focus on the practical aspects of your journey that will propel your spirit to expand and move forward. By envisioning the future of your dreams and focusing on each step, you will experience very little resistance. When you hold your vision, the present takes on a quality that allows you to move right into your future. Then it becomes quite clear what road to take, what door to walk through.

Here's a visualization you might want to try:

Imagine yourself communicating effortlessly with people every-where you go — on trains, at dinner parties, networking events. See yourself being at ease and confident about expressing who you are. The confidence is there, the freedom to express yourself is there, because you've done all your homework. You are unconquerable! You are able to enjoy these social settings, because this is where you can spread your wealth, your information, your love.

In order to begin to manifest your outreach, it is important to fol-low a plan, create a strategy you can adhere to that will help you stay organized and be most effective. The next three chapters will provide you with those steps, enable you to stay grounded and keep you moving ahead at the same time. We'll begin with the splash sheet.

THE SPLASH SHEET

When you begin to make your telephone calls to set up workshops or intro programs, to inquire about potential hosts and sponsors, the splash sheet can be a very handy tool. It is especially good for those of us who get tongue-tied while we're on the phone and don't want to forget any of the points we want to get across. I must confess, this happens to me quite a lot when I get excited — I notoriously forget half the things I've intended to say. The splash sheet saves me from relying on my memory and from many potentially embarrassing moments.

A splash sheet is like a script. It's a script you can read — or better yet, take your cues from — while you're on the phone. No one need ever know. Especially if you learn the material well enough so you don't sound like you're reading it off the page. You'd be surprised what people can hear on the phone — so don't forget to smile.

The splash sheet should contain all the pertinent points you want to discuss. Bullet the text, if you like, or write the sentences out in short paragraphs so they're easy for you to read. This way, instead of relying on your brain (a difficult task when you're nervous or feeling under the gun), you can use the splash sheet as a reminder.

On the next page is a sample splash sheet that Dr. Evan Fleischmann, N.D., used when contacting the Scarsdale Community Center. As you see, it is neat and easy to read. He used bullets and separated the information. He stated the need for his services up front and then backed it up with his education and experience. I especially like that he reminds himself to tell people that his presentations can be tailored to their needs.

SPLASH SHEET for Scarsdale Community Center
Planning and Choosing Your Dietary Supplements

- I am an expert in natural medicine
- Why you need me to present to your group
    - Over 60% of Americans use some form of alternative medicine
    - Your members are looking for truthful information about alternative medicine
    - Your members are concerned about drug side effects
    - Your members are probably taking supplements without proper guidance
    - Your members want to break free from dependence on medication

• The therapeutics NDs use	• The principles of naturopathic medicine
o Herbs	o First Do No Harm
o Homeopathy	o Identify and Treat the Cause
o Nutrition	o Doctor as Educator
o Counseling	o Prevention
o Energy medicine	o The Healing Power of Nature
o Education	o Treat the Whole Person
o Hydrotherapy	

- What is naturopathic medicine?
    - Naturopathic medicine is a blending of the traditional healing arts with modern medical science
- Naturopathic medicine can help people of all ages and both genders
- Naturopathic medicine is appropriate for acute and chronic care for all kinds of conditions
- Introducing myself as a practitioner
    - Degree from National College of Naturopathic Medicine
    - Practicing for over 5 years
    - Previous presentations and writings
        ◊ LBI Foundation of the Arts and Sciences, Loveladies, NJ
        ◊ Fall Wellness Fair, Chestnut Ridge, NY
        ◊ Spring Wellness Fair, Chestnut Ridge NY
        ◊ Vegetarian Times
    - Professional affiliations
        ◊ AANP
        ◊ NYANP
- Presentations can be tailored to your needs

Here are a few more pointers when using your splash sheet, from the book *How to Make a Million-Dollar First Impression,* by Lynda Goldman and Sandra Smyth.

Remember, the people you are speaking with on the phone:
- cannot see what you are wearing,
- do not see your office space,
- and only hear the words you use,
- but will hear if you are insecure
- and will know if you are smiling.

Another helpful tip I learned from this book changed the way I speak and listen to people on the phone.

The tip was: Adjust to each person's tone and mood as soon as possible. This is a very subtle practice, and one that can make a significant difference in the way a conversation proceeds. If the person on the other end of the phone has high energy, match their energy. If they speak slowly and quietly, do not try to overcompensate for their quiet energy by speaking exuberantly; try to match their energy without drowning the conversation. This is not about manipulating the conversation, it's about bonding energetically.

THE BLURB

Okay, you're on the phone with a prospective host, you've gotten their attention by introducing your idea for a workshop. Now they want you to send them some information about your course or presentation and they want to know more about you. The best thing to send them at this point is a *blurb.*

The blurb is a one- to two-page document that describes your workshop in detail. It conveys why the workshop is important to a particular audience, why the material is relevant, and why you are the person to present it. It is a synopsis of your presentation with an outline of the topics you will address.

Be sure to send the blurb soon after your phone conversation. If you wait too long, your host could forget about you altogether or decide to fill in the slot with a program by someone else who perhaps responded more promptly. As soon as you hang up the phone, create a cover letter that refers to the conversation you have just had, and then send them your blurb and your bio. By fax or e-mail, not by snail-mail.

Dr. Fleischmann wanted the Scarsdale Community Center to host his workshop entitled "Planning and Choosing Your Dietary Supplements." Here is a sample of the blurb he sent:

Planning and Choosing Your Dietary Supplements: Increasing Consumer Awareness
By Evan Fleischmann, N.D.

This two-hour workshop is intended to teach consumers the fundamentals of dietary supplement composition and selection. At completion of the presentation, participants will be able to make more confident and educated choices about dietary supplements.

Over 60 percent of the U.S. population uses some kind of alternative medicine, and American consumers are spending billions of dollars on dietary supplements each year. Most are basing their purchase decisions on what they hear and see in the media, and are frustrated because what they hear in the media keeps changing.

They want to know who the experts are that can guide them through the maze. They want to know who has the education and accurate unbiased information they need. There are so many brands and prices and choices when it comes to dietary supplements; how do consumers know that they're getting the right supplements at a fair price? They want to know: Do antacids really help osteoporosis?

Should I take capsules, or tablets? What is the proper dose? What is stearic acid anyway? What is the difference between brand names and generic or store brands?

Naturopathic physicians, the medical experts in alternative medicine, are the experts your members are looking for. This workshop will inform and empower your members to make educated choices.

Workshop Outline

- Vitamin A vs. beta-carotene
- Calcium
    - o Which form is best
    - o How much to take
- Vitamin C
    - o How much to take
    - o Which form is best
- Multivitamins
    - o One vs. more a day
        - Potency
        - Completeness
        - Size
- Vitamin E
    - o Natural vs. synthetic
    - o What are mixed tocopherols?
- Vitamin D
    - o How much to take
    - o Made with the help of sunlight
- Vitamin B12
    - o Sublingual vs. oral
- RDI / RDA
- Capsule, vegicap, softgel, tablet, powder
    - o What's the difference?
    - o Fillers, binders and sweeteners explained
- Cost vs. quality
- Herbs
    - o Tincture, capsule, tea
    - o Standardized or not
    - o Does brand matter?

In working with a potential sponsor for your presentation, stay flexible. If the organization is interested after receiving your blurb and they have only a two-hour slot to fill even though you know your course needs four hours — be flexible. Get your foot in the door. Present your workshop. When they see how wonderful your presentation is and how many people enjoyed it, they will ask you how much time you need for your presentation the next time.

When putting your blurb packet together to send to a prospective sponsor, remember:

- The first page you send will be the cover letter.
- The second page(s) will be the blurb.
- The third page will be your bio.

You might also want to attach a separate sheet of testimonials from people who have taken your workshop in the past.

THE FLYER

I used to have a recurring dream whenever I was involved in an event — whether it was my own or a client's. I'd imagine that I was in a helicopter, sitting in the open door, dropping flyers to the neighboring cities. I never wanted to miss anyone's house or place of business. My desire that everyone should know about the event I was promoting has always been so strong, even in my unconscious dream state, that my enthusiasm would push me out the door each day to pass out as many flyers as I could.

Anyone can distribute flyers around a neighborhood. But unless you have the enthusiasm and the energy behind the placement of these flyers, you might as well leave these pieces of paper (on which you've spent so much time and money) inside a nearby garbage can.

Because it is not about the pieces of paper you leave, it is the energy and enthusiasm with which you leave them.

IT'S ALL ABOUT ATTITUDE

For example: I paid two interns the same amount of money to distribute flyers for a yoga program in two different sections of the city. Samantha was very excited about the intro program that we were putting on because she was interested in hatha yoga and knew that if enough people came to the program, she would get a discount when she enrolled in the yoga course herself. Nancy, on the other hand, didn't have any interest in yoga; she just needed some extra money and agreed to help us pass out the flyers.

The night of the intro program, I asked people where they'd heard about the event. Some had heard about it on the radio, some had read about it in the newspaper. Twenty people showed up from the area where Samantha had distributed the flyers. Not one person showed up from the area where Nancy had passed them out.

When I spoke to Samantha after the event, I asked her if she knew why so many people from that area had come. She said, "Everywhere I went I talked to people about hatha yoga. Most of the people had never heard about it, so I explained to them how amazing it was for the body and how easy it was to learn. People would comment on how energetic I was and I guess they wanted to see if learning hatha yoga would give them more energy too."

You see, it's not about getting the job done. It's the attitude and enthusiasm you exude that attracts people to you and to an event.

So if you hire someone to represent you in accomplishing even the smallest of jobs, be selective. Make sure you know the attitude with which they are going to do the job.

Look at the difference it can make in the mere act of passing out flyers! Imagine the impact of an event when everyone working for the event comes from that space of enthusiasm.

MAKING AN EFFECTIVE FLYER

The flyer is a piece of paper that you hand someone, post for people to see, insert in a newspaper, or deliver to someone's mailbox or fax machine. It can come in various shapes and sizes and any range of sophistication. It may even include tear-offs or an order form.

The most important decision you will make about your flyer is where you post it. If it will be going in windows or being posted on walls or bulletin boards, your flyer should be big and bold and legible even at a distance. If you aren't sure where the flyers will be going, you may want to make two different versions: one as a handout, one for posting.

If you are planning to use tear-offs, a phone number is not enough. Use a couple of words in addition to the phone number. Otherwise, when your prospects do empty their bags, their wallets, or their purses, they'll wonder what this scrap of paper was about and throw it in the trash and you will lose your interested prospect.

Think about adding a stack of cards near the flyer or stacking several flyers together along with an invitation to take one.

Do not remove someone else's flyer from a bulletin board because it's in a prime spot. Remove only flyers that are outdated. If you find a large board, think about printing your flyer in different colors and placing a number of copies in different areas on the board. Be aware that every passing set of eyes sees them from a different height, so be sure, when you scatter your flyers, to place one high, one low, and one in the middle to accommodate people's levels of vision.

COST AND DESIGN

You can spend seven cents per flyer and make several copies or spend considerable less by printing originals from your own laser printer. The quality is higher than from photocopies, and shaded art or clip art will reproduce better. Whatever way you decide to go, be sure the flyer looks professional.

Usually flyers are either crowded with too much information or they're too skimpy and don't provide enough details. Unless you are a whiz with design programs, seek out a graphic designer and have them help you with the placement of the text, the mood and style of the piece. They know how a flyer should look. It's their job.

If you do go to a graphic designer affiliated with a printer, ask them about the price difference between offset printing and photo-copying. This may determine your decision.

White paper with black ink is clean and simple, but think about whether your flyer (depending on where you will be leaving it) would receive more attention if it were on colored paper. You can get solid colors in various hues: violet, green, deep red, fluorescent yellow . . . Whatever color you decide to use, think about what would be most appropriate for your audience. For instance, Kinko's has a pretty extensive selection and you can purchase as many sheets of paper as you want. You are not limited to producing your flyer in predetermined lot sizes of five hundred or a thousand.

There are many specialty stores now that sell only paper. I spend hours in these places, browsing for the best colors and textures if I'm promoting something very special. If you decide to purchase these expensive items, be sure the paper doesn't take away from your message. Some of these papers are so elaborate, they have the tendency to do just that.

A SPONSORED FLYER

If your event is being sponsored or hosted by another individual or organization, always place the presenting organization's name at the top of the flyer and the name of the event — the who, what, where, when — after. Using bullets provides readers with an eye-catching list of good reasons to attend, a list of benefits they will reap. Include the price, how people can reach you or the sponsoring organization, and how to register. And if you have room, include a little information on yourself. And always, always be sure to include the phone number for contact.

design for

impact

The Anthropology Department at Smith College

presents a lecture by

JOANNE EHRET

International
Acupuncturist/Chinese Medicine Specialist

Topic:

Chinese Medicine and Springtime Maladies:
Exploring a traditional paradigm of healing
to reframe and redefine asthma and allergies.

Thursday, April 27, 1995

7:00 - 8:30 pm

at the

Neilson Library Browsing Room
Smith College

Herbal Tea will be served.

*Joanne Ehret studied Acupuncture and Chinese Medicine at the Tri-State Institute of
Traditional Chinese Acupuncture in New York City and Chinese Herbal Medicine in
Beijing, China at the Xi Yuan Hospital of the Academy of Traditional Chinese Medicine.
She has taught acupuncture and Chinese Herbal Medicine since 1984 at the Tri-State
Institute and has a private practice in Northampton, MA specializing in internal medicine
(respiratory, digestive and gynecological disorders).*

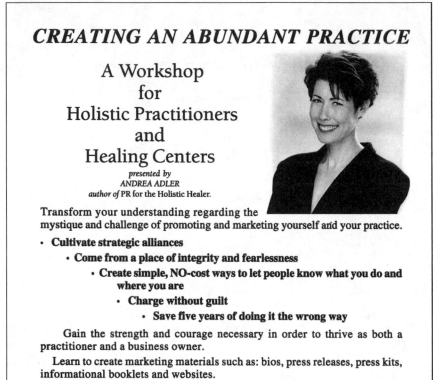

CREATING AN ABUNDANT PRACTICE

A Workshop
for
Holistic Practitioners
and
Healing Centers

presented by
ANDREA ADLER
author of PR for the Holistic Healer.

Transform your understanding regarding the mystique and challenge of promoting and marketing yourself and your practice.

- **Cultivate strategic alliances**
    - **Come from a place of integrity and fearlessness**
        - **Create simple, NO-cost ways to let people know what you do and where you are**
            - **Charge without guilt**
                - **Save five years of doing it the wrong way**

Gain the strength and courage necessary in order to thrive as both a practitioner and a business owner.

Learn to create marketing materials such as: bios, press releases, press kits, informational booklets and websites.

As we journey through the topics, you will understand the many promotional and marketing opportunities available to you in a way that will resonate with your own sense of integrity and purpose.

MOMENTUM STUDIO **SATURDAY, OCTOBER 26, 2002** **1:00 - 7:00 PM** **1807 Second Street. Studio 42, Santa Fe** **Price: $125**	CALL **505-983-7777** TO REGISTER AND FOR INFORMATION **www.HolisticPR.com**

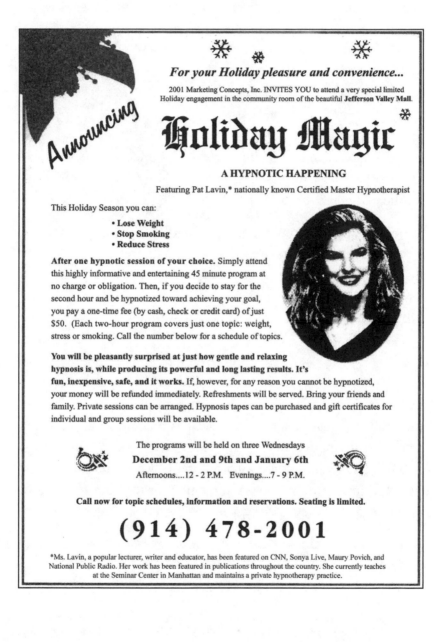

Think about where the flyers should be distributed. Certainly you will want to distribute them in areas that are geographically close to where your event will be present-ed. What about health-food stores, bookstores, spas, healing centers, cleaners', post offices, supermarkets, college book-stores, college cafeterias? Think about who your audience is and target the places they go.

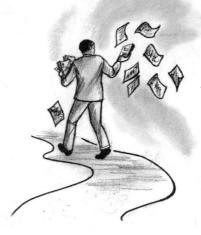

Don't be shy. Get out there and pass out those flyers! And while you're passing out those flyers, you might as well leave a few of your brochures.

THE INVITATION

Whether it's for an open house, a seasonal event, a ceremony or a friendly gathering, an invitation is a nice gesture and an age-old cour-tesy people still appreciate receiving. You can create an e-mail invita-tion, but I'd suggest sending a hard copy as well. This way, if your intended recipients never receive the e-mail or they are out of town and don't receive the hard copy, you've covered all your bases.

If you have the time and the ability to generate an invitation on your computer, by all means, do so. If you are not computer savvy or artistically inclined, here are a few suggestions:

1. Find a photo that depicts what the presentation is about and

scan it into your computer along with the text you've composed for the invitation.

2. If you don't have a scanner, take the photo to your local printer or ask a friend who owns a scanner to scan it in for you and print out a copy.

3. Ask your local printer to show you some sample invitations they've done in the past.

4. If you do not know how to use any of the graphic software available for computer, perhaps you have a friend who is an artist and would be willing to hand-draw your artwork. Take the drawing to the printer and ask them to copy the image onto the paper stock you've selected for your invitation. Then go home and print the text onto the same sheets.

There are plenty of Websites that offer artist images for a minimal cost. Try going to www.google.com and typing in *art websites* and see what comes up.

don't be shy ~

spread

your

wealth . . .

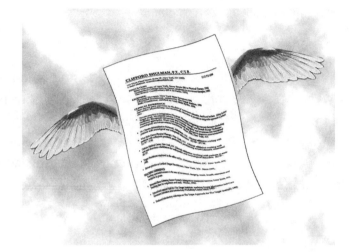

CHAPTER 11
RELEASING MATRIKA

Releasing Matrika

Now is the time for the world to know, your words are sacred.
~ Hafiz

Joy, oh, joy! You have a commitment from an organization that wants to host your event. You've collaborated with the program director and established an agreed-upon time and date. You're both excited to be working together and, of course, both parties would like an abundance of people to attend. In order to accomplish this goal and let the media, the people in your community, and the immediate universe know about this event, you will need to prepare a *press release*.

A press release is written primarily for the media. It is used to attract newspapers and TV and radio stations to write about you, or have you on their show, or interview you. It is your job to make this release crisp, informative, and interesting. If you take your time and do the release correctly, the press will see the value of your presentation and will feel impelled to inform the public — by writing an article. Believe me, there is no better, no cheaper advertising than having this kind of free exposure.

Depending on the organization you're working with, your sponsor may have their own formula for creating their press releases. They may have their own list of places where they send their releases on a regular basis. Don't forget, many organizations — for-profits as well as not-for-profits — put on events all the time. They may have their system down to a science. Why re-create the wheel? Ask them if they plan to write the release or if they'd like *you* to write it. If they want you to write one, ask them who they normally send their releases to. What newspapers? What radio stations? What TV stations? They may not hand over their list to you, but they may let you know verbally who their contacts are.

Even if they opt to send out the release on their own, you may want to send one of your own. Duplicating this effort is not a bad thing, because it ensures that the media receive the notification, but be sure to clear it with your sponsor or host if you decide to send one out in addition to theirs. They may want to see your rendition, to make sure it is written with the highest integrity or with a particular tone. They may also ask you to incorporate their logo.

Personally, I like to send my own releases to very specific newspapers, radio stations and local TV stations in the area. If the editors or journalists tell me they've received a release already, I ask them if they are planning to send a photographer and a reporter. Most likely the sponsoring organization will not be as persistent in this sort of outreach as I am. And if you've carefully coordinated your strategy with that of the sponsor, the fact that the media have received two releases may make the event look even more impressive.

After I make the initial contact and send the media my press release or other materials, I wait a couple of days and call the recipients back to make sure they've received what I've sent them and to see if they are able to attend. You can never do too much follow-up. The media like that you're on top of things. You may think you're being a pest, but you are simply doing your job — promoting your event.

THE ESSENTIALS OF A PRESS RELEASE

1. **The media do not like l-o-n-g releases,** so be sure to limit your text. Do not give them a detailed outline of your course or presentation, like you do on your blurb; it's not necessary. Provide them with "just the facts, ma'am," along with some interesting anecdotes, quotes, history and background. Depending on how much background information you i nclude about yourself in the release, you may or may not need to attach your bio.

2. **Make your press release newsworthy.** Make sure that what you write will be of interest to the readers of the publication that you are sending the release to. Keep in mind that reporters and editors love news stories with a human side to them. Make sure your story is entertaining, interesting, or newsworthy (hopefully all three). Otherwise, don't bother sending a release at all. Newspeople are extremely busy. They read hundreds of releases a day, seeking news to offer to their readers. So be sure your press release stands out and grabs their attention, especially in the first paragraph. Try to come up with an angle, a "hook" that will set your release apart.

3. **Target your release with precision.** There is no point in sending a press release about the opening of your new acupuncture practice to the editors of *Car & Driver* magazine . . . unless, perhaps, you have a story angle about stress-relieving exercises for drivers!

4. **Use the proper press-release format.** Construct your release in a manner that news professionals are accustomed

to receiving (see the basic press release format, on page 172). Make it easy for them to read and you will have a much better chance at getting noticed. And always, always check the press release for proper grammar and spelling.

5. **Write an excellent, compelling headline.** You only have a few precious seconds to catch the reader's attention. Make them count! The headline is 90 percent of your press release, and the primary goal of the headline is to ensure the rest of your release gets noticed.

Here are examples of headlines that illustrate that point:

LEGISLATORS GET GIANT RUBDOWN

This headline was used to describe a legislative event involving 40 massage therapists' giving simultaneous chair massages to various state senators and other politicians during Massage Therapy Awareness Week in Tallahassee, Florida.

SECRET TO BABY'S HAPPINESS FOUND IN DENVER!

This headline was used in a press release to inform the media of a demonstration of infant massage therapy techniques. Write headlines that attract attention, create feeling and paint a picture in the mind of the reader (think about the "photo opportunity"!). It is okay to put a comedic twist on your headlines to garner attention, but make sure the headline is real!

6. **Keep your press release concise.** Get to the point in the first paragraph — in fact, in the first sentence. Your story is likely to be ignored if you send a lengthy release that does not quickly state its purpose right up front. The first paragraph

should always answer the questions Who, What, When, Where, and Why — why is it important? Be sure your use clear, concise language and avoid using slang terms or exaggerated claims.

7. **Targeting is crucial:** Be careful whom you send your press release to. When compiling your own media list don't waste your time getting the e-mail addresses or fax numbers of every newspaper and magazine in the country — just the ones who
   would be interested in your story. Likewise, if you decide to purchase a media list, don't send your press release to every contact. Take some time to filter out the ones who wouldn't really care about your press release, no matter how good it is. Don't waste an editor's time with "clutter."

8. **Distribute your press release by fax, e-mail or snail-mail.** Just make sure you speak to the right person before you send it. Most of you will be dealing exclusively with the local media in your hometown. Get the names, addresses and contact information for all the local newspapers, radio stations, and television stations and begin there.

9. **When targeting a local television station, the person you must ask for is the *assignment editor*.** This is the person who assigns story ideas to the local reporters, and who subsequently will contact you for more details or to interview you or the subject you initially contacted them about. Usually you are confined to contacting your local ABC, CBS, NBC or Fox affiliate, as they are the stations that most often have a local news department. However, there may be other alternatives, including WB (Warner Brothers) affiliates, UPN (United

Paramount Network) affiliates, independent stations, or PBS
(Public Broadcasting System). For promoting awareness for
an event, most stations have a community calendar. Be sure to
contact every station in the area you are trying to reach. A
single mention of your cause or event has the potential to
reach hundreds, if not thousands, of viewers. If your message
is "soft news" as opposed to a major news event, you may
also try to get time on a local morning talk show or noon
news show, where stations often have more time to do more
community-oriented promotion.

10. **When targeting a radio station, your approach must be
    specific.** Unless you are targeting a news station, you should
    make an attempt to know the format and personalities at
    the station you are seeking coverage from. If your event is
    aligned with the type of audience a particular radio station
    reaches, you will have a much better chance at receiving
    publicity. For example, if you were performing free chair
    massages at the Country Hoedown Festival, your best bet
    would be to contact the local country-music radio tation.

11. **To target newspaper coverage, the same holds true.**
    There are many different departments within a newspaper. It
    is important you target the ones most appropriate, or your
    news release will no doubt end up in the wastebasket. If you
    are a massage therapist who performs sports massage, you
    may want to think about soliciting a story from the sports
    editor. If you want to be quoted as an authority in stress
    management in the workplace, you might consider contacting
    the business editor. If you are seeking coverage of your
    practice's ability to perform and teach infant massage,
    consider contacting the lifestyle or features editor.

THE BASIC PRESS RELEASE FORMAT

FOR IMMEDIATE RELEASE

For further information contact:
Full name of contact
Direct phone number
Headline

City, date (e.g., March 7, 2000):

- Introductory paragraph that answers Who, What, Where, When, and So What?

- A second paragraph offering more information on the cause or event you are trying to get coverage of.

- The third paragraph includes a quote attributed to somebody important, for example: "BioFreeze is a revolution ary product," says Joe Smith, owner of Healing Hands Massage Company, Inc.

- The fourth paragraph includes some more information, per haps another quote. This paragraph often includes history and background information about the company or person.

Sample press releases are found on the pages that follow..

NEWS RELEASE

Body of Truth. The Place for Whole Health.

For Immediate Release   August 15, 2001

Contact: Jenny Fox   845-331-1178

A CORNUCOPIA OF SURPRISES AT BODY OF TRUTH'S
FIRST ANNIVERSARY OPEN HOUSE

Kingston, NY - Body of Truth, LLC, the most comprehensive integrative health-care spa in the mid-Hudson region, will celebrate their first anniversary Open House Saturday, September 15, from 10:00 am to 4:30 pm. Located at 737 East Chester Street Bypass, Kingston, NY, Body of Truth will be offering FREE mini-treatments, samples, demonstrations, lectures, tours, refreshments and multitudes of good company.

Owned and operated by Simone Harari, Body of Truth, LLC was developed to be a prototype of what health care could be like in the future — an environment that is magical for both clients and practitioners. In keeping with this mission, guests remove their shoes upon entering. They are greeted by a floor-to-ceiling copper fountain, light music, subtle aromatherapy scents diffused into the air, exquisite Feng Shui design, and a warm, welcoming staff.

"Our intention was and is to create an environment that embodies truth, wisdom, and the kind of sanctity that provides options for people," Simone Harari says, "not just for the patient/client community but for the medical community as well. Doctors understand that there are many ways to heal and assist the human body to heal itself. So they refer clients to us to complement their patients' health-care needs."   Besides the in-house array of offerings, Body of Truth has alliances with the medical community, Lamaze teachers, La Leche League, and the Benedictine Hospital, where tailor-made classes are presented to their maternity and delivery unit. "We are looking forward to working with other local not-for-profits in the area," states Jenny Fox, administrative director; "we're also planning to open our doors twice a year to the community — for no charge — in order for everyone, regardless of income, to learn more about holistic health. Everyone is welcome to our Open House. We look forward to meeting our neighbors and unveiling a few surprises."

Photo opportunities are available all evening and individual interviews can be arranged with Simone Harari by calling Jenny Fox at 845-331-1178.

NEWS RELEASE
Florida State Massage Therapy Association
Established 1939
The oldest professional massage therapy association in existence.

For Immediate Release   July 5, 2000
Contact: Ron Scirrotto   (561) 882-0066
Jose Fernandez/Dan Grief,   (407) 628-2772
Chumney & Assoc.

HORSES GETTING RUBBED THE RIGHT WAY

Orlando, FL - The Florida State Massage Therapy Association is bringing two equine massage experts to Orlando this weekend to demonstrate the new science of therapeutic massage therapy for horses to its statewide members. These demonstrations will be held at the Radisson Hotel Universal Studios Orlando, 5780 Major Boulevard, on Friday, July 6, from 9:00 am to noon and from 2:00 to 4:00 pm. The demonstrations are part of the annual gathering of the association's members.

Don Doran, a third-generation horseman and licensed massage therapist, created the first equine sports massage (ESM) training program in the country after studying human athletes and comparing their muscle groups and other factors to those of horses. His program is designed to show how to prevent injuries common in athletic horses. Injury treatment, recovery and rehabilitation, including the use of "Equi-pressure," an acupressure course for horses developed by Doran, will be discussed during a hands-on demonstration of equine sports massage on Friday at 2:00 pm. "I actually worked with the University of Florida's sports-massage program for the human swim and track teams to help correlate human and equine athletic injuries," stated Doran. "Now people travel from all over the world to learn these techniques," he added.

The morning session will be conducted by Gayle Mya Breman, L.M.T., M.S.W., N.C.T.M.B., of the Upledger Institute. Through deomnonstation and lecture, Ms. Breman will focus on the application of delicate craniosacral therapy techniques to improve the health and well-being of horses. The prevalence of horse enthusiasts in central Florida should make both these topics of keen interest to a wide audience.

Photo opportunities are available all day on Friday, and individual interviews can be arranged with either speaker, as well as with Ron Stephens, President of the Florida State Massage Therapy Association. To arrange an interview, please call Jose Fernandez or Dan Grief at (407) 628-2772. or call Ron Scirrotto at (561) 882-0066.

For Immediate Release
April 1, 2002

Contact: Vicki Whitcomb   (413) 586-9594

The Anthropology Department
at Smith College presents
INTERNATIONAL ACUPUNCTURIST
JOANNE EHRET
Chinese Medicine and Springtime Maladies:
Exploring a traditional paradigm of healing to reframe an
redefine asthma and allergies

Northampton, MA: With allergy season looming, Northampton resident and international acupuncturist / Chinese medicine specialist Joanne Ehret wants to educate the community on complementary approaches to these bothersome springtime maladies. Joanne's presentation will be held on Thursday, April 27, 2002, from 7:00 to 8:30 pm at the Nielsen Library, Smith College.

Acupuncture uses fine, sterile needles to activate Qi (energy) in the meridians to maximize a complete circulation of energy. Acupuncture allows the body and emotions to release stress so that normal functioning can resume. "Small magnets are sometimes taped to acupuncture points in place of needles," Ehret explains, "a technique often used for children and adults who have needle phobia."

Frustrated with Western medicine's lack of effectiveness and its attention and treatment to only parts of the body and not the "whole body," Ehret became interested in the vast network of meridians — the energy channels of acupuncture — and their innate ability to link all parts of the body together. "By maintaining this 'human electricity' and its proper flow," Ehret states, "many illnesses can be prevented.)

A graduate of the Tri-State Institute of Traditional Chinese Acupuncture in Stamford, Connecticut, Ehret continued her studies in Chinese medicine at the Xi Yuan Hospital in Beijing as well as at the hospital's Advanced Clinical Course in Chinese medicine. These experiences nourished the initiative for the acupuncture and Chinese -medicine clinic where Ehret currently specializes in internal medicine, with a special focus on respiratory, digestive and gynecological disorders.

Photo sessions and interviews will be available. To schedule, ask for Vicki Whitcomb at (413) 586-9594.

IN SUMMARY

Choose the media most likely to carry your press release. Select those that carry similar write-ups on a regular basis.

Use the proper press-release form, complete with a headline that will attract the attention of the editor or reporter who will be deciding whether or not to use your item.

Direct your release to the appropriate person and include his or her name on a cover letter. It pays to call ahead to find out the name (and its correct spelling) of the person you should be sending your press release to. Call them and let them know your release is forthcoming. Then send the release and follow it up later with a phone call to make sure they received it and to find out if they have any questions you might be able to answer for them.

Be sure your press release does not contain typographical errors or misspelled words. Always send an original — not a photocopy — from your computer or typewriter, on professional-looking letterhead or news-release paper, if possible. The same holds true if you are faxing your release: use an original so that it transmits clearly to the recipient. And when your item is used as a newsworthy notice, send a thank-you note or call the editor in person to thank him or her for using your press release.

Do not call or write an editor demanding to know why he or she did not use your release for a story. Just let it go and try again next time. Contemplate why you think they didn't run it. Many factors go into determining which stories are used or not used, and those factors can vary greatly on a day-to-day basis. Always be polite and friendly. If you burn a bridge, you greatly reduce your chances of having subsequent story submissions picked up by that media source.

If you do get a great story that makes an impact on your event, you may think about sending the editor a thank-you note with a complimentary massage or an invitation to your healing center.

The press can be your best allies. But like most people, they don't like to be used or abused. By fostering a relationship with someone you connect with and building the friendship slowly, as with all relationships, it will be a long and beneficial one. Pace yourself with all media. Don't bombard them with every little piece of new information. Save them for the big-ticket items. Then they will want to hear about your progress, they will want to support your growth — by writing about you.

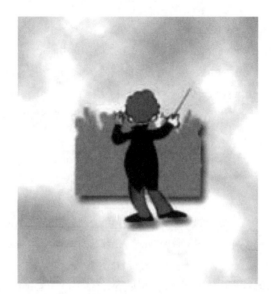

CHAPTER 12

ORCHESTRATING YOUR OUTREACH

Orchestrating Your Outreach

We are the music makers, and we are the dreamers of the dream.
Wandering by lone sea breakers, and sitting by desolate streams.
World losers and world forsakers, for whom the pale moon gleams.
Yet we are movers and the shakers of the world forever it seems.

~ Arthur O'Shaunessey

THE PRESS PACKAGE

The *press package* consolidates all your materials into a nice, neat parcel. Most of the time it's sufficient to hand someone your card or your brochure. But there will be times, particularly when the media are involved, that you'll want to hand them a press packet for their perusal.

It's not necessary that you have this package together right away. It's something that you build slowly and meticulously while you go about your daily business. When articles are written about you or when you write articles or columns yourself, when you receive any kind of recognition or attention from the press, when you have testimonials from clients about your good work, this is the vehicle through which you can showcase your achievements. The more events and workshops you present, the more panels and speaking engagements you have, the fuller this package will become. Once again, this is something you don't need right away. But do consider it for the near future, and include the following:

- a cover letter, if you are sending your package addressed to someone specific;
- your brochure;
- a bio;
- a press release, if you have one;
- your latest flyer (for an upcoming event);
- articles written about you;
- articles written by you;
- testimonials;
- your photo;
- your card, inserted in the slot provided by most presentation folders.

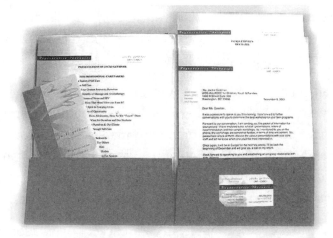

Jacki Gethner has one of the most impressive press packages I've ever laid eyes on. The soft green tones are easy on the eyes and the imagery of fingers and hands is so inviting, you want to read her materials immediately to find out what she does. By using the same image of hands that she uses on her brochure, and on her letterhead, she creates a theme that invites the reader to move through the package easily.

Jacki does not include her resumé in this package — nor should you, in this instance, as it is not appropriate. Your audience is not interested in details, only in the broad picture of who you are and what you have accomplished.

WHY DO YOU NEED A PRESS PACKAGE?

The press package can be useful when the media are interested in interviewing you or writing about you. It gives them background to chew on. It might also be just the ticket you need when a potential host or sponsor is interested in partnering with you. The press package shows interested parties that you are organized, that you take pride in your work, that you have a history and that you have interesting aspects to your profession they may not have been aware of.

You can begin the creation of your press package by purchasing a nice heavy-stock or plastic folder that has pockets. You can spend a lot of money and have folders printed to match your stationery, your brochure and your card. You can have all kinds of fancy graphics that might cost an arm and a leg — or you can create one that is simple, elegant and inexpensive.

One way to achieve continuity in your packet presentation without spending a lot of money is by creating a logo that goes on your card, on your stationery and on your brochure. You can also have a sticker made, using the same logo to place on the folder cover, giving it visual interest. When your card, your brochure and your press package all match, it looks like you have taken the time to design your marketing materials, and people respond to that kind of care.

You can also find loads of meaningful photos or images to place on the cover by doing a little research. Just don't overdo it — keep it simple.

HAVE A PHOTO OF YOURSELF

There are three reasons to have a photo of yourself on hand and current:

1. To include in your press package;
2. To hand to the media if they ask for it;
3. To provide a sponsoring organization with one to place beside your bio in their calendar or newsletter.

It used to be that the press preferred a black-and-white photo with submissions to their magazine or newspaper. They would request a specific size, too, as it made their job easier and it was less expensive to print. But nowadays, with access to scanning machines and sophisticated computers, one can submit color or black-and-white photos to these establishments and the size is no longer an issue.

There are many options to having your photo taken: you can ask a friend who has experience taking "head shots"; you can call photography studios and compare prices; you can find a local establishment where they take passport photos. Personally, I would suggest investing in a good head shot by a professional as you'll be able to use this photo on your brochure, for the media, for many things that come up — for at least five years.

Whatever route you decide to take, make sure the photo represents what you look like in the most positive light, and be sure that it looks professional. Once you decide who will take your photo, be sure to have about twenty-five copies filed away at all times.

TIMING THE OUTREACH

What good is all your hard work to put on a great event if you haven't given your audience enough time to schedule it on their calendars? If no one comes, if no one's heard about it in time?

There have been millions of presentations that have gone sour because people haven't allowed enough time for their campaign. Thousands of dollars are wasted every day on events because strategies are not planned out properly or the necessary exposure isn't scheduled appropriately. All this money, all this time might have been better spent climbing a twenty-four-story building in the poor section of town and throwing dollar bills out the window. At least the people catching the bills would have benefited from the waste.

Once you have your blurb, the bio, the press release, the flyer, your invitations, be sure to give yourself **one full month** to:

- send out the invitations,
- notify the press,
- distribute flyers,
- make follow-up phone calls.

During that month: Call newspapers in the area where the event will be held and find out to whom you should send the press release, the flyer or the blurb for the weekly calendar or community section. Every newspaper has this section. They are obliged to inform the community of local events, whether an event is free or not. And they should, if they are doing their job properly, welcome your contribution.

While you're on the phone with the calendar person, ask to speak to a reporter whose stories feature health issues. Talk to the reporter about who you are and what your event is about. Ask them if they wouldn't mind if you sent them some information. Then, in addition to sending your materials to the calendar section, send the reporter your press release and flyer.

INTERNS

If you discover that you have less time than you thought for gathering lists, making phone calls and passing out flyers, you might want to consider placing an ad for an intern.

Interns can be extremely helpful. One of the things they can do is call local radio and TV stations for you and try to get you an interview. Besides, it's more professional when someone calls the media on your behalf. It places you in another category, it creates more of an intrigue and provides you with a healthier distance than if you were to make the calls yourself. Interns can be a great asset in this case and in other ways, as well. They can help you:

- distribute flyers;
- gather phone numbers and e-mail addresses of organizations;
- make initial calls to get contact information;
- call newspapers to find out the name of the person to whom they should fax the flyer and blurb for the calendar or community section;
- surf the Web for strategic partners — partners who may want you to write an article for their Website or participate in a chat, or who may even want to sponsor one of your workshops;
- register people, welcome people, and help pass out handouts at the event.

There are many competent college students anxious to work for a relatively small amount of income, just to receive the work experience. When I was living in Massachusetts, every office I walked into had interns. Some offices had between two and ten interns working for them. True, Amherst and Northampton were small towns, college towns, where transportation was not an issue and there were lots of students available. Still, while your area may not seem so luxuriantly endowed, there are colleges and high schools everywhere.

Call around to schools and colleges nearby and ask to speak to a guidance counselor or the placement office. Instructors and counselors are thrilled to pass on job opportunities to their students. Students' parents are happy that their children are making money, the students are happy to learn and be able to place the experience on their resumé.

The placement or counseling office may ask you to write up a small ad on a three-by-five card describing the intern's responsibilities. Ask them how they'd like it sent (e-mail, fax) and then send it over immediately while they still have you on their mind. Once you start interviewing a few students for the intern position, as with your ever-ready PR materials, keep a contact list of available interns on hand.

PREPARING FOR THE EVENT

Make sure you are as thorough and meticulous in the presentation of your event as you are in the materials that you create for it. Feel secure. Do all the necessary research, be prepared. Learn your material inside out, upside down and sideways. You can't be too familiar with your content.

When I'm preparing a talk, I read my speech out loud in front of a mirror, I read it into a tape recorder, I practice it with friends and relatives. I take it with me on my daily walk. I go over it and over it until all I need are a few sheets of paper lined with bullets to remind me of where I am on the page and where I need to go next. You want to be able to walk into that room filled with people, with confidence — and the only way you can do that is by knowing your material inside out and knowing that you have everything you need. So create a checklist for yourself and begin early to get these items together days before the event. Do not wait until the last minute. Whatever the type of event you are presenting, these are the essentials:

- guest book
- sign-in sheet for the press
- name tags
- handouts
- your brochures
- extra pens and paper for taking notes
- the questionnaire (see page 193)
- snacks
- drinks
- music
- flyers announcing the next workshop
- cash box, if necessary
- receipts, if necessary

Always bring extra everything, just in case you run out. The less you have to leave until the last minute the better. You'll have plenty of other things to think about as the time grows closer to the event.

THE DAY OF THE EVENT

The big day has arrived. The day you've been planning for, for months. What is your state of mind before you walk out of your home? How are you feeling? How are your nerves? You can attend the event frazzled and out of control, nervous, thinking that everything that could go wrong will go wrong — or you can enter the room feeling confident that everything will be magnificent. The choice is entirely up to you, as it always is. However, there are preparations that will help ease you through the process. Here are a few to consider before you leave your house.

1. **Meditate.** Find a quiet spot on the floor or in a comfortable chair and sit quietly for a few minutes. Breathe deeply and begin to let go of all your thoughts. Just watch them as if they were a movie playing out in front of you. Do not become attached to any one thought. Focus your attention quietly on your breath. Begin to watch the in-breath and the out-breath as if they were waves moving on their own without any force or will on your part.

   Just let your attention rest without effort on your breath. Once you notice that your breath has slowed down and you have relaxed into your body, begin to see yourself in the room in which you will soon be presenting, welcoming people. See and feel yourself rooted in your body, enjoying each and every person who greets you. Staying open-hearted and in the moment frees you from anxiety.

   Now, slowly, see yourself moving over to the podium or to the center of the room where you will begin your presentation. Before you say a word, look around, see all the beautiful faces in the room. Take in their curiosity, their delight in being there. Inhale the warmth and love that permates the room and then welcome everyone to the program.

This type of visualization is a precious tool. I use it every time I'm asked to speak. Seeing myself in the room, visualizing myself as calm and collected, relaxed and open, helps me to fully imbibe that state. In that state other states can't coexist; there's literally no room for fright or the jitters.

2. **Go over your speech or presentation.** Take your notes and stand in front of a mirror and recite your talk from beginning to end. Then, do it again. Be sure to allow your introduction, your welcome to segue smoothly into the first part of your talk. I've found that once I'm totally secure with the very beginning of my presentation, the rest of it pretty much flows on its own.

3. **Go over your checklist**. Make sure you check off all the things you need to bring with you as well as all the things other people are supposed to bring. Make calls if you need to double-check. You can never be too sure or too prepared. And besides, this is about you feeling absolutely secure today. So do whatever you need to, to have that experience.

4. **Wear something that makes you feel rooted and in your body.** Don't wear anything too tight, anything that would inhibit you from moving around freely. Don't wear anything too revealing; this too could hinder you from feeling comfortable.

Think about a color that will give you confidence and make you feel at ease. Bright reds and oranges make you feel more outgoing and fiery. Blue is calming, green engages the intellect, violet or purple supports the throat and communication center.

5. **Eat something light,** so you don't feel famished when you get there, even if food is being served. A little food is grounding and sustains your energy level on an even keel.

6. **Arrive early.** The earlier you are, the more confident you'll feel, the more in charge, the more balanced. And this way, you'll have time to set up the room the way you want it.

7. **At your venue, take a good look around** and see where you want to place the chairs, the tables, the lights, the music. Make sure there is room for a registration table, a table for handouts, plenty of space between the seats for your guests. If you need a podium, microphone, VCR, TV monitor or overhead projector, you'll be there early enough to set things up before your guests arrive.

8. **Your intern or assistants can help you.** Have them register people at the door, invite participants to sign your guest book, give out literature (your brochures, handouts for the course, information on upcoming workshops and courses), distribute press packets to the press and have them sign the sign-in sheet, walk enrollees to their seats, serve tea, cookies, or other refreshments and see that guests are comfortable.

9. **Be sure that you and your hosts make people feel welcome** when they walk into the room, and throughout the presentation.

10. **When guests arrive, gently suggest they sign your guest book.** Have them print their name, address, telephone number, and e-mail address in the book. This will be a great resource to you later when you decide to do a mailing or want to promote your next workshop.

11. **Use this event to announce your next class, your next seminar, your new book.** Have flyers available that refer to upcoming events, or a calendar. This way, your audience knows you are constantly making appearances in various locations and can pass this information on to their friends.

12. **The time is here.** Everyone is in their seats. Continue to remember what you experienced in your visualization: see and feel yourself rooted in your body, enjoying each and every person you meet. Before you speak, look around, see all the beautiful faces in the room. As you did in your vision, take in their curiosity, take in their delight in being there. Do it for real, here, now. Inhale the warmth and love that permeates the room, welcome everyone to the program . . . and now begin.

13. **When you have finished your presentation,** it's a nice gesture to thank those people who helped you with the event. Gratitude is contagious: it's a wonderful, positive energy to spread around.

14. **Before you conclude and break to the informal after-event opportunity,** talking to all the people who will inevitably want to talk to you, ask everyone in the room if they would please fill out a small questionnaire before they leave.

THE QUESTIONNAIRE

The feedback questionnaire is a document that you present at the end of your workshop. It's an excellent fact-finder and will provide you with answers to questions you normally wouldn't arrive at any other way. For instance, you wouldn't know that the woman in the blue dress sitting in the front row is from a local hospital looking for presenters to speak about complementary medicine, would you? You wouldn't know that the man in the second row is an MD looking for a Reiki practitioner for his office twice a week. You wouldn't know that the man in the suit standing by the watercooler is from the Arthritis Foundation and wants a massage therapist to work with his patients, would you?

This is the beauty of the questionnaire.

It also becomes a vehicle through which you can ask specific questions to learn about other workshops people may want in the future. And when you look back at a later date to see who is interested in what specific workshop, the questionnaire becomes a significant reminder.

In your questionnaire, be sure to include the statement "Please comment on the workshop." These responses can become testimonials for you to use in your marketing packet later. Those comments will also show you where your presentation is strong and where you need more work. I have provided a sample questionnaire on the next page.

SAMPLE QUESTIONNAIRE

Please fill out this questionnaire before you leave. The information will help us improve the workshop and accommodate your future needs.

Your name _____
Organization _____
Occupation _____
Type of business _____
Address _____
Phone and fax numbers _____
E-mail address _____

What did you enjoy about the presentation?
_____
_____

What would you like to see changed?
_____
_____

Would you be interested in having (*your name here*) present this program at your organization? _____

If so, who would the contact person be?_____

Phone number? _____

List topics you'd be interested in hearing more about:
_____
_____

How did you hear about this presentation?_____

Your comments on the workshop:
_____
_____
_____

Please hand this back to a person at the registration desk. Thank you!

We hope you enjoyed the evening.

THE DAY AFTER THE EVENT

All your hard work, all your loving attention to every single detail has brought you to this moment and to the wonderful sense of satisfaction you must be feeling. All the sacrifices you have made before and during the event — quality time with your children, cooking for your family, getting to the laundry, getting to the dishes — now seem like a dream, a dream with a happy ending. Your family is proud, your friends are proud. People responded favorably to your presentation. Everyone who attended was interested in what you had to say. How do you feel? You should feel great! Go celebrate! Relax! Give yourself a day off. And while you're sitting by the pool or relaxing in the hot tub enjoying a nice tall glass of iced tea, take a few moments and evaluate what happened.

Take your time to reflect and really think about each of the following questions:

What did *you* like about the event?

_____

_____

_____

_____

_____

What went smoothly?

_____

_____

_____

_____

_____

What needed more time and care?

_____

_____

_____

_____

_____

What would you have done differently?

_____

_____

_____

_____

What would you keep the same?

_____

_____

_____

_____

After you have answered these questions for yourself, gather all the questionnaires that people completed at your event and take a close look at their responses. Is there synergy between what you experienced and what your audience experienced? You may want to make a mental note of this, even write these thoughts down to remember for your next presentation.

Then, follow up on all the leads you were given. Call back those people who stated they were interested in wanting a presentation. These leads may take you toward more speaking opportunities, panel presentations, consultations, more clients. Have your intern call the press people who attended your event and ask them if and when an article will be coming out.

When you have collected all the newspaper articles that were written about your glorious event, cut them neatly out of the newspaper or magazine and make Xerox copies. Be sure you have the name of each newspaper and the date visible on each copy. Then, include them in your press package. You may even want to laminate the original, so it doesn't discolor. By laminating, you preserve the newspaper print and are assured of good copies in the future.

rejoice . . .

relax . . .

reflect . . .

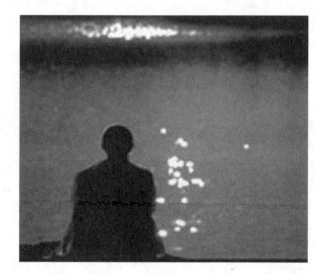

CHAPTER 13

COMPOSING YOUR THOUGHTS

Composing Your Thoughts

When you speak, your words echo only across the hall.
But when you write, your words echo down the ages.

~ Bud Gardner, coauthor,
Chicken Soup for the Writer's Soul

There are numerous ways you can let your clients know that you care about them, above and beyond seeing them on a regular basis and offering them your personal expertise. You can provide them with an occasional gift certificate, or a monthly or bimonthly newsletter that brings them up to date on your new courses, workshops, seminars, and books that will enhance their health. A newsletter can be a powerful tool.

THINK ABOUT AN ON-LINE NEWSLETTER

An on-line newsletter costs less than one you mail, it is instantaneous, and it can include color and other graphics features that would be incredibly costly in hard copy. Here are two examples of people who have created on-line newsletters and who have had wonderful success distributing them to those they wish to reach.

Marilyn Gordon, director of the Center for Hypnotherapy, located in the Bay Area, began communicating with her audience by sending out postcards to her mailing list each month announcing her workshops and programs. She tells us:

As costs rose and our mailing list grew, we decided to take a look at other options. I'd received other newsletters by e-mail, and I knew I wanted to create one that was visually stunning as well as informative. One day I received an e-mail ad from a company that offered special easy online software for newsletters and announcements, to which we could add our own pictures, paintings, and other graphics. I was attracted to the fact that it was inexpensive, easy and potentially beautiful.

We took all our e-mail addresses and fed them into the database, and we created a monthly newsletter with wonderful colors and great artwork. We also included articles about our work, announcements of our products, courses, and workshops. We've had some thrilling feedback. "I love your newsletter. Please keep me on the list." "Thanks so much for sending those messages. I find them so helpful, and I love the artwork." "Sign me up!" "Send me one of those!"

On our homepage, we have a special sign-up area for new people to subscribe. We've collected names from people who've called us for information from our print ads or from referrals or from our client base. It now costs us $25 per month via the Web, compared to $400 per month via the post office. Don't worry, we still give the post office our business in other ways, but we now have a means to reach people via cyberspace, which provides a wonderful alternative.

Marilyn says that through her newsletter, she has sold more products, enrolled more people in her classes and workshops, and has reached more clients with her services.

A SELF -PRODUCED NEWSLETTER

Jeremy Nash, an executive coach and speaker, and director of Communication at Work, LLC, decided to send out his on-line newsletter twice a month without using a service. He created his e-mail newsletter in order to be in regular communication with existing and prospective clients.

Whenever, I'm attending a networking function and meet people, I ask for their card and ask their permission to send the newsletter to them.

Sharing my ideas and suggestions has always felt like a natural way to reach people, push the envelope of my own thinking and provoke others to think, as well. It appeals to me much more than calling people directly.

On several occasions I've bumped into people I'd met many months earlier, and they've told me how much they appreciate getting the newsletter. This positive feedback has helped me keep my faith alive that I'm truly building a practice that will ultimately impact many thousands of people in a profound way.

And through his on-line newsletter, more people have signed up for Jeremy's speaking circles and programs.

HARDCOPY NEWSLETTER

Some months ago, Patricia Karnowski sent her green-hued newsletter, *The Barefoot Acupuncturist,* to a number of residents in New York's Westchester area. While still living in New York, I had the good fortune to receive one. I had no idea how she got my address, but when I received this lighthearted, colorful, informative newsletter, I thought, "This is the best thing since George Foreman's lean machine."

I called her soon after and praised her for her ingenuity. Where had the idea come from, I asked her, to start this newsletter? This is what she had to say:

I decided to put out a newsletter when I arrived in Westchester County as a licensed acupuncturist with a masters degree in Oriental Medicine. I needed to get my practice going quickly, as I was basically broke after spending the better part of a year and all of my savings traveling around the country. I took stock of the area and realized that even though I was only about 30 minutes outside of New York City most people had no idea what Oriental Medicine was or how it fit into health care. I must admit that I'd had no idea of the depth or breadth of this ancient medicine myself, until I spent more than four years studying it full time.

I designed my newsletter as a tool to educate the community about acupuncture and Oriental Medicine. I feel that as a practitioner in the United States in this early part of the 21st century it is my responsibility to educate people. Whether they use this medicine or not, they need to have a basic understanding of what it is. I'm not sure how else they could make informed decisions. I am the expert in the area, so I feel that it is my duty to take this on.

My newsletter is filled with the latest research and what is happening in the field on the legal front both locally and nationally, in addition to answering the basic questions of what it is and how it can be used. Of course I also include all of my credentials.

I started developing my list of who to send it to by looking in the yellow pages and holistic directories. I picked out anyone I thought would care to know about Oriental Medicine or acupuncture, like yoga teachers, massage therapists, psychotherapists and people working with the elderly. I also sent it to other acupuncturists in the area to let them know that I'm here in case they would want to refer patients to me. I use my newsletter as part of a packet I put together, with a personal cover letter and my curriculum vitae, to take along with some fresh-baked cookies (from Sam's Club, I have to admit) to doctors' offices to introduce myself as the new acupuncturist in the area. After I've spoken with them, I add them to my list. I also put stacks of of the newsletter at health-food stores or any other place that will take them.

I started getting patients immediately as the result of these newsletters . In the first seven months I grossed around $40,000 with no other advertising (I was broke, remember).

Patricia's newsletter is one of the finest examples of making an offering — educating, informing with humor — that I know of.

THINK ABOUT WRITING THAT BOOK

Writing and publishing my own book not only helped me to define and refine myself in terms of what I had to offer; it gave me the confidence to author and publish the second edition of this book. I had been approached by a large publishing company to bring out this second edition, an offer many first-time authors would love to say they've received. But I had so much fun marketing and promoting my first book, I wanted to do it again.

Self-publishing is also, in the long run, more remunerative. With this second edition, I'll be printing twice the number of copies, setting up distribution arrangements with outside vendors, catalogues, and schools, and linking to a range of Websites. In addition to just selling books, the potential it opens up for invitations to present workshops and speeches, for participating on panel discussions, traveling to places you would never be able to afford to go to otherwise, is so much greater. Writing a book helped me to attract corporate sponsors, and will soon become the catalyst for starting a TV show. To say writing a book is worth the time and effort we put into is, well, putting it mildly.

Here are a few testimonials from *Turbocharge Your Consulting Business Now,* by Elsom Eldridge, Jr. and Mark L. Eldridge. As you will read, John Conrad Levinson and Linda Pinson have both benefited immensely from writing a book:

My personal experience with book writing is mind-boggling. Someone once asked me how much I made for my first Guerrilla Marketing book. The answer I gave was $10 million. The book itself only paid me about $35,000 in royalties, but the speaking engagements, spinoff books, newsletters, columns, boot camps, consulting, and wide-open doors resulted in the remaining $9,965,000. If any consultant wants to open wide the doors to a myriad of opportunities, my suggestion is: write a good book!

~ Jay Conrad Levinson,
Guerilla Marketing International,
the father and author of *Guerilla Marketing*

Writing and publishing a book is a great starting point if you want to be considered an expert in your industry . . . but it is only the beginning. The key is to write a good book that is better in some way than those already written on the subject and then to market it in every way possible. In 1986, I was advised that it was fruitless to write another business planning book. Sixteen years later, the "fruitless" book, Anatomy of a Business Plan, 5th edition, is still on the market and has helped more than a million business owners through the process of writing a business plan. Listen to yourself and follow your vision.

~ Linda Pinson,
*Out of Your Mind and Into the Marketplace:
Helping Entrepreneurs Through the Business
of Doing Business*

YOUR THOUGHTS AND EXPERIENCES MATTER

I cannot emphasize enough the importance of writing a book. You will be amazed at how easily and effortlessly doors fling open when people know you are an author, especially when the book is well written and valuable to a particular audience. In addition, the media love to write about people who have authored a book. Why? Because they like to interview people who know what they're talking about. They like to interview people who are experts in their field and who are passionate enough about something to put it on paper. They love to tell their audience there is information available on a subject they know their audience will be interested in: "Boy, do we have news for you." "So-and-so will be on our show today to give you the top ten tips on how to . . ." "Read all about So-and-so in our newspaper." The media do a great job promoting your book for you. All you have to do is give them something informative to brag about.

By writing a book and defining yourself as an expert you,
- increase your visibility and prestige;
- enhance your credentials;
- raise your income;
- give yourself exposure, which leads to more opportunities.

Why not begin today to document your thoughts, your observations and your experiences? Remember, there is no competition. No one will ever write a book that covers all the material you have to share. Your experiences are your experiences.

A SIMPLE WAY TO BEGIN

One way to initiate the process is to purchase a two- or three-hole notebook binder and place three pieces of paper inside. On the first page, write down as chapter headings all the topics you'd like to write about. Then select one topic from the list and start writing about that topic. When you have a sufficient amount of written material, insert the data into your computer and print it out. Insert those pages in the binder and put in three more pieces of paper. Select another topic from your list of chapter headings and repeat the procedure.

When you have written and printed out all the pages, read them over. Does it flow? Is it clear? Is the energy sustained, or are there places where it drops? Is the tone inviting? Edit the places where editing is needed. Input the rewrites into the computer, edit some more, and print out the pages.

Carry the binder around with you, everywhere. This way, when you're in a bus or a train or waiting for an appointment, you can begin to elaborate and fill in the pages of each chapter. Before you know it, you'll have written several chapters and you won't be able to stop writing. All the information that you've accumulated over the years will begin to pour out of you like a stream of fresh water. Let it flow. Try not to edit your writing at the beginning. Just keep it moving through you.

WRITING, MORE TIPS

Dan Poynter, author of *The Self-Publishing Manual,* makes the following suggestions:

When you're at home writing, and you have a myriad of other things that need to be done, don't be afraid to combine projects: do some writing and then go water the lawn.

Do more writing, and clean a room in your house.

Return to writing, and then clean another room. It actually stimulates the brain when you take these breaks, and you end up accomplishing more.

When you feel confident about what you're written, send each chapter to a person you know is an expert regarding this particular chapter — for peer review. Ask them to review what you've written and send it back to you as soon as possible; you may want to give them a time frame for responding to you. Their input is invaluable: they will critique your writing and perhaps add more substance, give you insights into the chapter you never thought about before. They may even find an error or two that you'll be able to fix in plenty of time. Their feedback may be hard to swallow at first, but the best writers accept criticism wherever they can, as long as it's relevant, and are willing to eliminate or change sections where their writing doesn't work or they haven't thought something all the way through.

If you cannot write your book because of limitations with your physical vision or other issues, create a team of support, or perhaps offer to do an exchange with a writer; writers love receiving bodywork. Just think of the writing as an extension of your learning process — all those papers and research projects you wrote in college or in your professional training. There are also voice-recognition computer programs available that you can speak into. This software is still fairly new, but is quite accurate and will automatically type your words on the screen. A client of mine uses this program all the time and loves it.

If you have decided to focus only on the writing of your book and seek out a publisher or an agent to represent you, you will need to create a book proposal. The proposal can be written before the book is completed. Depending on the material, there are agents who will be satisfied with a proposal, a bio, the table of contents, and one or two sample chapters.

THE PROPOSAL

A proposal is a synopsis of a book. It summarizes why the book is necessary at this time and for what readership. As you write your proposal, you will want to be very clear as to who the readers will be, why there is a ready-made demand for this book, and why you are the person to write it.

The proposal not only defines your target audience, it becomes a carrot, so to speak, to help you secure an agent (if you decide to go the agent route). Some people send their proposal straight to publishers, others have agents who send it for them. Some people have contacts at publishing houses and don't need to create a proposal at all.

While in the midst of writing my first book, *PR for the Holistic Healer,* I thought I'd wanted a publishing house to produce my book. So, I sat down and wrote the following proposal. I had an agent at the time and she asked me to write a proposal for her to send out to potential publishers. In the end, I decided to publish the book myself. But I was asked to write a proposal and was glad I did. It helped me define my audience as well as my mission and convinced me once again of the importance of following through on this project — in case I had any idea of giving up before it was completed.

You can find many more proposals in the book *How to Write a Book Proposal,* by Jeff Herman. Here's a sample of my first book proposal to give an idea as to how one looks and a sense of the kind of research that is needed.

PROPOSAL FOR
PR FOR THE HOLISTIC HEALER:
A Handbook on Promoting and Marketing Your Practice
by Andrea Adler

OVERVIEW

According to *The New England Journal of Medicine,* 425 million visits were made in 1993 alone to practitioners of "alternative" or "complementary" therapies — representing $13.7 billion in expenditures. Now, seven years later, that number has doubled. Earthmed.com, an on-line holistic and lifestyle community, has over 100,000 practitioners in their directory. Onebody.com, another on-line holistic Website, delivers services, networks, publishes, and sells products to the 33-billion-dollar complementary health-care market. They also have a directory with over 70,000 practitioners. Attached is a list of other sites with even more staggering figures.

These only prove that the use of alternative or complementary healing methods is not just a fad, but the beginning of a tidal wave. They also tell the story of our present and our future: people are seeking alternative ways of healing, and spending billions of dollars to get them. If we have millions of people spending all these dollars, who are they visiting? They are visiting practitioners, lots of them, many of whom have minimal experience running a healing business.

Furthermore, the majority of these healers are not provided with the tools that will help them succeed in the business world. Many of these skilled healers graduate from school without realizing that in addition to healing the mind, body and spirit, there is the issue of building their practice. To do this involves self-promotion, marketing and the foundations of sound financial practice. Even those who have been in the marketplace for several years and are experiencing growing pains need to rekindle their knowledge of how to promote and market themselves. With the increasing numbers of practitioners moving into the mainstream (acupuncturists, Reiki healers, massage therapists, breathworkers, chiropractors, homeopaths) the time is ripe for *PR for the Holistic Healer: A Handbook on Promoting and Marketing Your Practice.*

MARKET STUDY

A cursory search on Amazon.com revealed that there are over 4,000 books on the topic of public relations. There are books of a general nature like *Guerilla Marketing Handbook* by Jay Con Levinson, textbooks, government-related books, and hundreds of other PR titles that target a specific industry. *Making the News: A Guide for Nonprofits and Activists,* by Jason Salzman, is the only title that could possibly have any relevance to this audience, proving this is an untapped market.

VOICE AND SCOPE

PR for the Holistic Healer: A Handbook on Promoting and Marketing Your Practice targets the healing population, providing them with a step-by-step guide on how to garner publicity, generate partnerships and cultivate media exposure. It will be used as a reference and will help healers gain the strength and courage necessary in order to thrive as both a healer and a business owner.

Because this population, many times, has difficulty identifying themselves as businesspeople, this book speaks directly to this ambivalence. Rather than keeping these two aspects of healer and businessperson separate, *PR for the Holistic Healer* will help healers to integrate these two perspectives, thereby creating harmony and balance.

The style is friendly, straightforward, supportive. There is a warm, nonthreatening approach that helps the practitioner walk through the self-exploratory exercises. Each practitioner, whether fresh out of school or a seasoned healer, will understand the importance of creating the perfect resumé, the perfect bio, the perfect sound bite. Healers will learn how to articulate and define a clear sense of themselves; how to differentiate their healing methods from others', how to create positive paradigms, and how to build strong relationships with existing institutions.

CHAPTER BREAKDOWN:

INTRODUCTION

PART 1:   THE INWARD JOURNEY
- The Beloved Resumé
- The Bio
- The Sound Bite
- The Business Card
- The Brochure
- Exploring your Inner Circle

PART II: GATHERING THE NUGGETS
- The Priceless Offering
- Money and Your Practice
- The Power of the Word
- The Subtext of Enthusiasm
- Your Practice Is Bigger Than Others Believe It to Be
- Back tothe Lists
- Contact Sheet
- Strategic Alliances
- Sponsorships
- Agreement
- Internet Possibilities

PART III: ABOUT YOUR PRACTICE
- Your Physical Space
- Your Psychic Space
- Competition — and the Fact That There Is None

PART IV: THE OUTWARD JOURNEY
- The Splash Sheet
- The Blurb
- The Press Release
- The Flyer
- The Invitation
- The Photo
- The Press Package
- Timing the Outreach
- Interns
- Before the Event
- The Day of the Event
- The Questionnaire
- The Day After the Event
- Think About Writing That Book
- The Proposal
- A Few Closing Remarks
- Acknowledgments

Throughout the chapters, healers will be shown how to customize the information to suit their particular needs. Sample bios, resumés, press releases and questionnaires will be included to help healers prepare for jobs and meet prospective partners, as well as understand how, why, and when to create workshops, presentations, and other events.

Firsthand anecdotes and practical advice will help healers navigate unexpected or difficult situations. Self-evaluation tools will help them pinpoint and realize their career and lifestyle goals.

As healers journey through this book, they will have an understanding of the promotional and marketing opportunities available to them in a way that will resonate with their own sense of integrity and purpose. They will discover, at their own pace, exactly how these tools apply to them, how they can take advantage of these opportunities and how they can implement them in their life and in their practice.

CREDENTIALS

Andrea Adler, the author, has the experience and enthusiasm to reach out to this distinctive audience. Her love and respect for healers, coupled with her extensive PR and marketing background, make her the perfect author to reveal the strategies that have been the basis for her successful career.

Ms. Adler has been a marketing and public relations consultant for over 15 years. From 1993 to 1997, she owned her own public relations firm in Amherst, Massachusetts, where 90 percent of her clients were healers (see article enclosed). Prior to that, she promoted and marketed not-for-profit organizations and artistic ventures in the Catskill region of New York. Ms. Adler moved to Westchester, New York in 1997 and has since worked as a PR consultant for corporations from law firms to Internet companies.

A dynamic motivational speaker, Ms. Adler has conducted workshops for business professionals, healing centers and professional associations. She has led seminars at political gatherings, business establishments, and in public and private schools.

An accomplished writer, Ms. Adler has written videos for the American Film Institute and for corporate clients. She has written articles for *Body Mind Spirit* magazine, *The Times Herald Record,* and *Uno Mismo,* a New Age magazine published in Buenos Aires. Ms. Adler wrote Herbal Life's first audio promotional tape, and fund-raising collateral for Bread for the World, EDF (Environmental Defense Fund), City Harvest, Food for Thought, Co-op America, and other not-for-profits. She is completing her first novel, *Pushing Upward,* a spiritual coming-of-age story, in addition to *PR for the Holistic Healer: Promoting and Marketing Your Practice.*

PROMOTION

Ms. Adler has already been asked to speak, write articles and create chats on the Internet for Blue Horizons (a community for holistic practitioners), ForHealers.com, the Learning Annex, GirlsInc., and PR Forum for PRSA (Public Relations Society of America).

Ms. Adler will be presenting her workshop *PR for the Holistic Healer: A Workshop on Promoting and Marketing Your Practice* to the following organizations this year: the Professional Healing Network, the Learning Annex, GirlsInc., PR Forum for PRSA (Public Relations Society of America), the Katonah Healing Arts Alliance, The Greenhouse, Mirabai Books of Woodstock, Wainwright House, the Florida Massage Therapy Association (FSMTA), the Sarasota School of Massage, Tools for Life, and the Academy of Chinese Healing Arts.

Each of these engagements will present an opportunity for Ms. Adler to market her book. Because of her PR expertise, she will have easy access to TV shows and radio shows that target this audience as well.

WHERE WILL THIS BOOK BE SOLD?

Mainstream bookstore chains
New Age/spiritual bookstores
Internet sites
Massage Therapy Journal

Spirituality and Health
Yogajournal.com
ForHealers.com
Reiki.org
Earthmed.com
Onebody.com
Oxygen.com
Freeagent.com
Newagejournal.com
The Trager Institute
Acupuncture Society of New York
The National Commission for the Certification of
     Acupuncture and Oriental Medicine
Esalen Institute
The Swedish Institute
Kripalu
Omega Institute
Hippocrates
Wainwright House
Florida Massage Therapy Association
Sarasota School of Massage Therapy
Tools for Life
Academy of Chinese Healing Arts

WHO WILL BUY THIS BOOK?

Healing centers
Professional associations
Wholesalers that sell to practitioners
Health-food stores throughout the U.S.
Practitioners who are graduating from training centers
Practitioners who are affiliated with healing centers

Practitioners who participate in workshops at healing centers
Practitioners who are members of associations
Practitioners who read New Age magazines and participate
     in their Websites
Practitioners who frequent New Age bookstores and
     health-food stores
Practitioners who watch New Age talk shows
Practitioners who listen to New Age radio shows
Practitioners who tell other healers

Do understand that every proposal is unique, just as every book and every topic is unique. It is important that you research your topic and find other proposals to use as samples. Be sure you are clear yourself on the audience you want to target.

There is a wonderful resource book written specifically for writers called *The Writer's Guide to Book Editors, Publishers and Literary Agents,* also by Jeff Herman. The book is quite hefty and comes out annually, providing writers with names and addresses of hundreds of agents, editors and publishers — some of whom may be very interested in your material. It also describes in detail how to write a book proposal, be it for fiction or nonfiction.

If you decide to go the self-publishing route, I'd highly recommend purchasing *The Self-Publishing Manual* by Dan Poynter, www.parapublishing.com. This book is by far the best manual ever written on self-publishing and helped me tremendously to publish my first and second book. I'd suggest reading this book about ten times — no, maybe twelve times. Read it over and over until you've learned everything there is to learn from each and every page. And then, read it again to make sure you didn't forget anything. The people I've spoken with who have followed Dan's suggestions are now very successful authors and publishers. It may be too early to determine the ultimate sales of this book that you hold in your hand.

*The process of writing itself
will gift both you and your reader.
For as you continually invoke the powers
of words and expression, and call upon your
inner guidance and wisdom, your book will
reflect your state of expansion.
Your growing sense of awareness,
of certainty, of enthusiasm,
will be conveyed to the reader.*

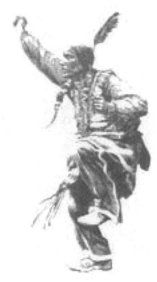

CHAPTER 14

COURAGE

Courage

*Wake up to your inner courage
and become steeped in divine contentment.*

~ Gurumayi Chidvilasananda

I was done with this book. All the writing had been completed, the illustrations were ready to be inserted and it was about to be sent off to the printer. And then I met a man, on a airplane going to Tucson, who talked to me about his software company and how scared he was to leave the comfortable, well-paying job he had worked at for six years, to pursue his dream — a dream he had thought about for ten years. I saw how much courage it took him to confront his family about this huge transition he was about to make. And as he spoke to me, it reconnected me with my own courage, made me mindful all over again of the courage it takes for practitioners to follow their dreams.

After thinking about this for a few days and holding up production on the book, I knew it was a chapter I had to include before you really dove in. Because the reality is — even if you have envisioned your future in the most minute detail, even if you are able to see yourself as whole and have integrated every exercise in this book into your being — unless you wake up to your inner courage, there is a good chance you will remain stuck and allow insecurity and fear to maintain its grip on your life.

True courage, I have come to experience, is an inside job that takes diligence and fortitude, patience and love. When my heart, my head and my will are all in agreement with respect to my next move — I move. I don't wait. I have learned to trust that connection when it happens.

This connection creates a subtle knowingness, an inner strength that gives me the awareness that what I have to say and the actions I perform will be in sync with the highest good. Whatever move I make, because of this alignment, has a postivie result.

Think, for a moment, about a time when you were scared to death to do something. But you wanted that something so bad that you were willing to take the leap and go for it. How did you feel after you leapt? Pretty content, right? (Unless it was the wrong thing to leap for). Well, the more you trust yourself to take those leaps, knowing that you have connected with your heart, your head and your will, the more contentment you will feel, and the less fear you will experience in your life.

Courage is a muscle that needs to be exerciseed – just like our brains.

If I hadn't experienced this transformation from fear to courage myself and created the necessary vehicles to get myself "out there," I wouldn't be able to sit here and write these words with such conviction.

I cannot count the number of times I'd thought about giving up writing and presenting workshops to practitioners. I mean, all I kept hearing was "I have no money," "I can't afford a book or a workshop!" "Won't you give me a discount or allow me to take the workshop for free?" Wherever I went, the city, the state, the country, it made no difference; it was the same scenario. Practitioners are embracing such tools today, but even two years ago, few saw this information or these skills as an important and worthwhile investment in their career.

I couldn't help but think, "What the hell am I doing, busting my behind, hardly able to feed or clothe myself, pay my own bills? Wouldn't I be better off expending all this energy on something else — like another vocation?"

And then, I'd hear this little voice inside say, "Have faith, be patient." The voice was hardly discernible. During the day, I'd have to block out all the sounds and distractions to hear it, but while I was meditating, sitting quietly and peacefully in my meditation room where no outside noises could be heard, the voice was loud and clear. I wouldn't be able to ignore it.

And then there'd be an e-mail from someone thanking me for writing my book, asking if they could purchase another copy for a friend, or I'd get a call from a practitioner asking for a consultation because they were beside themselves with confusion. The signs were all there, and they remain a significant part of my evolution.

True courage
must stem from the depths of our being.

Having the courage to listen to that voice that speaks to us in the quiet spaces of our hearts separates true seeking from pretense. When we ignore or put off that voice, we only delay the process of our own movement, a process that we cannot — and dare not — sidestep. It was, I believe, Anais Nin who said that at a certain point the price we pay for sitting on our own courage, our own integrity in action, becomes higher than the price of action, even in the face of potential failure.

*Courage is about taking the initiative
to be conscious, all the time, to the thoughts
that run our lives —
and to the possibility of freedom.*

Even beyond matrika shakti, the power of the word — the power of what we say and how we say it — there is the discipline of listening to our thoughts and distinguishing the quality of energy they carry. We don't need to dwell on the ones that bring us down or instill fear. We have the choice at all times, every minute of our waking state, to pick and choose the thoughts we want as companions. And it is those companions that can turn us into warriors.

*Making the decision
moment by moment to choose uplifting thoughts
— the ones that take us, and those around us,
to a higher destination —
transforms us into warriors.*

When people feel our passion energetically, they step back and see us in a new light. They feel the weight of our conviction, and when we speak they listen. We are amazed at the courage within ourselves. And, slowly, we begin to get used to it and actually learn to enjoy it. We may even begin to expect it.

I am fully aware that taking the first step can demand every ounce of courage you possess. I will not pretend for one minute that it's not the toughest, most monumental thing in the world to do. Whether it's making that first call to a potential sponsor, composing a brochure, or contacting a physician to present your modality, taking that first step is a milestone! And even if it does not feel easier, there's a forward movement, an energy, that begins to carry you through.

Then, all of a sudden, you'll see, you'll be on this roll and you won't be able to stop yourself. The momentum and excitement of receiving your first YES will turn you into a marketing enthusiast, and that's when the magic begins. Your very core will be quivering with excitement, not fear, and that enthusiasm will carry you through every phone call, every e-mail, every interaction that you approach. The contentment that comes from having made that leap is absolutely priceless, and indescribable.

Trust your inner courage. Watch your thoughts. Be the warrior, and become steeped in divine contentment.

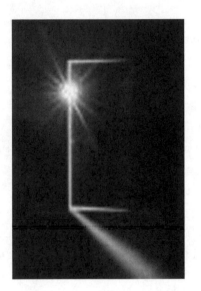

CHAPTER 15

IN CLOSING:
CHOOSING INTEGRITY

In Closing: Choosing Integrity

*Your work is to discover your work
and then with all your heart to give yourself to it.*
~ Buddha, the *Dhammapada*

I have shared whatever knowledge I could with you regarding thejourney of creating abundance in your practice. I purposely have not gone into the purely financial aspect of the business (taxes, deductions, reimbursements) because I prefer to focus on the internal and external manifestations of thought and action. I want to get into the essence, into the heart and soul of how practitioners and healing centers can create abundance, rather than venturing into the "strictly business" arena of expertise.

There are plenty of accountants and financial advisors who can be of help to you in these areas. When it comes time to needing this kind of assistance, and we all do at some point, ask a friend or a peer if they can refer a financial specialist to you. Look in the yellow pages and call these professionals — interview them, determine for yourself which advisor resonates with your sensibilities.

I've wanted to share my own experience as well as people's stories, because that's how I learn best. Besides, if I were to write about reimbursements, for instance, and what is being discussed at this moment on the state and national level, it would be ludicrous. The laws are changing so fast that by the time this book comes out, the issues will all be different.

Now that you have completed the journey through these pages, I do hope that as you move through your life and experience the fruits of your practice, you remember what is most important. And that is: the work you do on yourself — how you treat others; how you evolve on your own individual path. It is only through this self-effort that we able to reach higher and higher states of consciousness. Only through this sort of process do we instinctively become more sensitive to ourselves and to those around us; then we attract those people whom we want in our lives and draw to us the people we want to work with. Only then will we enjoy a success not merely of monetary fulfillment, but of a genuine sense of great peace and joy.

The more respectful and caring you become toward those you serve, the more you will create the magical buzz you are yearning to — naturally, unselfconsciously — and that buzz will spread like wildflowers. And then, one day, all you'll have to do is open your door, greet all the clients wanting your skills, and enjoy the abundance that will effortlessly pour into your life. It will flow like a golden stream, and such divine beings as Lakshmi, the goddess of wealth, will open the palm of their hand and grant you the prosperity you have earned. The abundance of a livelihood that sustains you, that connects you to a world of wonder and awe, that offers you the joy of growth through service and doing what you love.

So please remember:

- Never stop working on yourself.
- Live consciously.
- Stay open.
- Dissolve your ego, or at least set it aside, while you are doing your work.
- Allow people to be where they are without judgment.
- Remain humble.
- Respect the knowledge that you have acquired, share it, nurture it.
- Constantly evaluate your motives.
- Stop comparing yourself to others. Everyone is unique. Discover what works for you and then act on that understanding — passionately.
- Charge appropriately, fairly, for your service.

I would like to close as we began, with an offering –– in this case, an offering of inspiration, or words that have carried me forward in my own journey. These words are from a speech Nelson Mandela recited on the day he was inaugurated as president of his nation, in 1994. When I first heard these words, I became incredibly moved by their potency and even now, every time I read them, they rekindle an energy inside me, a force that I try to sustain. These words have helped me to see my role in the universe more distinctly. They have helped me to dissolve my own fears and have inspired me to spread my own wings a little wider. I hope they inspire you to spread yours.

Our deepest fear is not that we are inadequate.

Our deepest fear is that we are powerful beyond measure.

It is our light, not our darkness, that most frightens us.

We ask ourselves,

Who am I to be brilliant, gorgeous, talented, fabulous?

Actually, who are we not to be?

You are a child of God.

Your playing small doesn't serve the world.

There's nothing enlightened about shrinking so that

other people won't feel insecure around you.

You were born to make manifest the glory of

God that is within you.

It's not just in some of us; it is in everyone.

And as we let our own light shine,

we unconsciously give other people permission to do the same.

As we're liberated from our own fear,

our presence automatically liberates others.

Your life work is a work of art.

A craft to be most carefully mastered.

For patience has replaced time.

And you are your own destination.

~ author unknown

ACKNOWLEDGMENTS

There are times in your life when you know you're doing the right thing. When people show up you haven't seen in years or people you've just met help you for no good reason — when the red carpet rolls out beneath your feet and all of sudden everything in your life falls into place. Well, that's what happened while writing both the first and second editions of this book. It was surreal how friends, strangers and relatives came from nowhere and supported me with their time, their talents and their suggestions. The following are just a few of the people I'd like to thank for their faith in me, for all their support, their dedication and their love.

Thank you . . .

Brian Adler — for being the rock.

Cynthia Briggs — my dear friend. Thank you for your wisdom and laser-beam editing. Thank you for your "above and beyond the call of duty" *seva* and for helping me become a better writer with each book I write.

Gene Krackehl — for reminding me that love and friendship are the most important part of the path and for being such an exquisite example. Thank you for your magnificent cover, once again.

Joanne Ehret — for the use of your resumé and bio and for the great adventure you let me share with you.

Michael Crouch — for understanding how to play the game and having the heart and wisdom to play it.

Ron Scirrotto of Chumney & Associates — for your contribution to the chapter on the Press Release.

Joe Lubow, Pat Lavin, Charles Jones, Marilyn Gordon, Jeremy Nash, Patricia Karnowski, Linda Frank — for your work in the world and for your contributions.

Cliff Shulman — for allowing me to share your stories with others. You are the finest example of everything I have tried to communicate in this book.

Ti Caine — for being the light at the end of the deep, dark tunnel I sometimes had to crawl through.

Marie Harris — for opening you arms and your heart and gifting me with your house, your car, your computer and your cats.

Bill and Diane Sileo — two of the most loving, caring persons in the universe. Thank you for your generous hospitality.

Elizabeth Pinson — my soul sister. Thank you for your unending love and support.

Aysha Griffin — for coming through at the last minute with the photo.

Carmine Puma — for your friendship and loyalty.

Ann Marie Eastburn — for your illustrations.

Evan Fleischmann — for being there — with everything.

Dan Poynter — for writing *The Self-Publishing Manual.* Your book will go down in the archives as being the best written, most informative book on self-publishing — ever.

Particia Bragg — for being your authentic self.

Melanie Pablemann — For giving and giving and giving your design expertise. This book would never have been made without you.

To Gurumayi Chidvilasananda, to Baba and to the Siddha masters — who watched over me and gave me the strength to pursue my dream.

To all the practitioners and healing centers who have shown interest in my work and in my books — may you all flourish with tremendous abundance.

Blessings to you all!

To my sponsors,

who provided me

with their faith and trust,

and the means through which

I could bring this book

to the world.

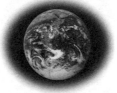

Supporting
Your Success

At BIOTONE, we applaude your continued commitment to promoting and educating others on the benefits of massage therapy.

Like you, we know how important it is to spread the message of health and well-being. Through our contributions funding massage research, ongoing support of community outreach and education, and development of innovative massage lubricants and spa products, we strive to touch you and your clients in a positive way.

Whether your are just beginning your career, or have many years experience healing others, you can count on BIOTONE to support your success and help you become increasingly valuable to your clients and the health community. Please call us for company and product information.

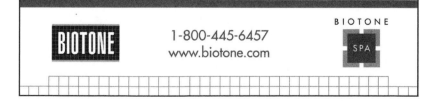

BIOTONE

1-800-445-6457
www.biotone.com

BIOTONE
SPA

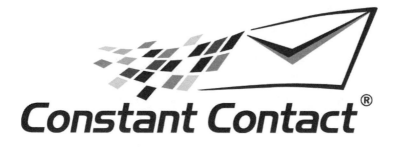

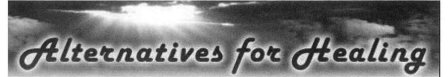

Alternatives for Healing

We are a national directory for the holistic therapeutic community. We advertise in over ten national magazines with a circulation of over 1.3 million readers. Plus, we are submitted in over thirty internet search engines. Because of our unique marketing efforts, we are able to significantly increase traffic to our website and to your business.

Other categories we include on our website are books, magazines, seminars, conventions and schools.

By advertising with us, any classes or seminars you offer are **included at no additional cost. Mention Holistic-PR and you will receive a special advertising discount.**

For further information call

Sonja Torres at (949) 322-3444
www.AlternativesforHealing.com

Let us help you be successful!

To all who share the quest
for the essence of well-being –
May your path be blessed with

abun-dance
and joy

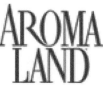

AROMA
LAND

Exclusive offer
for "Creating an Abundant Practice" readers :
35% discount if you enter "1029957261"
as your coupon code on the online order form.
Free shipping on orders over $45.00.

800.933.5267
www.aromaland.com

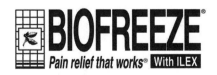

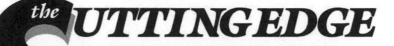

This book was printed and manufactured at

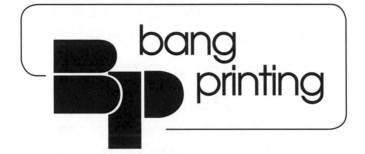

in Brainerd, Minnesota

For more information contact us at:
www.bangprinting.com
1-800-328-0450

REFERENCES & LINKS

Ti Caine, FutureVisioning
(www.ticaine.com)

Lenedra J.Carroll
The Architecture of All Abundance: Creating a Successful Life in the Material World
Published by New World Library, Novato, CA
ISBN 1-57731-189-2
333 pages, $24.00
1-866-284-3343
(www.LenedraJCarroll.com)

Gurumayi Chidvilasananda
Courage and Contentment: A Collection of Talks on Spiritual and Life
Published by SYDA Foundation
ISBN 0-911307-77-X
182 pages, $12.95
1-888-422-3334
www.siddhayoga.org

Paul E. Dennsion, PhD, and Gail E. Dennison
Brain Gym: Simple Activities for Whole-Brain Learning
Published by Edu-Kinesthetics, Inc.
Copyright 1986
40 pages
1-800-356-2109

Ann Marie Eastburn, illustrator, murals
Just Imagine, . . . Murals
PO Box 51954
Albuquerque, NM 87181
505-275-9251

Evan Fleischmann, N.D.
The Holistic Healing Center
747 Chestnut Ridge Road
Chestnut Ridge, NY 10977
845-425-5233
evan@EvanFleischmannND.com
(www.EvanFleischmannND.com)

Jacki Gethner, LMT-CADC 1
Regenerative Therapies
PO Box 11208
Portland, OR 97211-0208
503-287-3620
E-mail jackigethner@earthlink.net
(http://home.earthlink.net/~jackigethner)

Lynda Goldman and Sandra Smythe
How to Make a Million-Dollar First Impression
Published by GSBC
ISBN 0-9694996-1-2
164 pages, $15.95
(www.goldmansmythe.com)

Marilyn Gordon
Center for Hypnotherapy
1-800 398-0034
(www.hypnotherapycenter.com)

Richard Strozzi Heckler
Holding the Center
Published by Frog, Ltd.
ISBN 1-883319-54-4
131 pages, $12.95
(www.ranchstrozzi.com)

Shel Horowitz
Grassroots Marketing: Getting Noticed in a Noisy World
Published by Chelsea Green Publishing
ISBN 1-890132-68-3
306 pages, $22.95
1-800-683-WORD
(www.frugalmarketing.com)

Robert Moss
Dreaming True: How to Dream Your Future
and Change Your Life for the Better
Published by Pocket Books, a division of Simon & Schuster
ISBN 0-671-78530-3
351 pages, $14.95
Fax: 518- 274-0506

Jeremy Nash, Executive Coach
Communication at Work, LLC
914-762-0322
(www.clear-purpose.com)

Melanie Pahlmann
Lucid Design Studios Web Design and Desktop Publishing
505-982-6606
design@luciddesignstudios.com
(www.luciddesignstudios.com)

Dan Poynter
The Self-Publishing Manual
Published by ParaPublishing
Santa Barbara, California
ISBN 1-56860-063-1
421 pages, $19.95
(www.parapublishing.com)

Dan Poynter
Successful Non-fiction: Tips and Inspiration for Getting Published
Published by Parapublishing
ISBN 1-56860-061-5
142 pages, $14.95
(www.parapublishing.com)

Emanuel Rosen
The Anatomy of Buzz: How to Create Word of mouth Marketing,
Published by Doubleday
ISBN 0-385-49667-2
303 pages, $24.95
(www.emanuel-rosen.com)

Sherri Senné, Information on right-brain/left-brain function taken from *Creative Alternatives for a Changing World* offered by Creative Alternatives, PO Box 250, Palmdale, FL 33944, USA
(www.laffslearningarts.com)

Cherie M. Sohen-Moe
Business Mastery: A Guide for Creating a Fulfilling, Thriving Business and Keeping It Successful
Published by Sohnen-Moe Associates
 ISBN 0-9621265-4-3
448 pages, $24.95
(www.sohnen-moe.com)

ANDREA'S OFFERINGS

Andrea's presentations are both interactive and experiential. Participants quickly become motivated, excited about the future they are about to create, and Andrea provides them with the strategy to get there.

If your school, center, organization or professional institution is interested in having Andrea speak or present any of her workshops, e-mail:

andreapr@aol.com

If you are interested in attending or sponsoring a workshop, let us know. All you need is 10 or more people interested in the same workshop. It can be hosted in someone's home, office, healing center, business, school or any suitable location.

There is a good chance we may be doing a seminar or workshop in your area. Check our Website for workshop schedules:

www.HolisticPR.com

The following is a description of Andrea's current workshop series.

THE WORKSHOP
CREATING AN ABUNDANT PRACTICE

An eight-hour workshop designed for practitioners of all modalities that can be presented in three separate workshops. This course brings Andrea's book Creating An Abundant Practice alive, as practitioners are able to transform their understanding regarding the mystique and challenge of promoting and marketing themselves and their practice.

It will provide them with a step-by-step approach on how to garner publicity, generate partnerships and cultivate media exposure from a spiritual and practical perspective, and in a way that resonates with their own sense of integrity and purpose.

Marketing materials such as press releases, bios, informational booklets, brochures, cards, and newsletters will be discussed in detail, breaking through the obstacles practitioners face when preparing these materials.

Improvisational theater games will be introduced to help practitioners learn to act and react from a place of strength and confidence.

The games become a catalyst for letting go of outdated habits, guards, and inhibitions as we explore new ways to present ourselves. As a result, participants become more agile and flexible. They begin to trust instinctively that the choices they make are the right ones — for every situation.

INDIVIDUAL WORKSHOPS

The eight-hour workshop is availble as a series of three workshops. Please feel free to mix and match any of them to fit your specific needs:

Creating an Abundant Practice,
Marketing Materials for an Abundant Practice,
and Ignite the Spark of Creativity

CREATING AN ABUNDANT PRACTICE

A four-hour workshop designed for practitioners of all modalities. This workshop is an overview of the eight-hour workshop

As practitioners journey through the topics, they will understand the many promotional and marketing opportunities available to them in a way that will resonate with their own sense of integrity and purpose.

This workshop is usually presented in conjunction with the following two:

MARKETING MATERIALS
FOR AN ABUNDANT PRACTICE

This four-hour workshop focuses specifically on marketing materials: the business card, the brochure, flyers, newsletters, postcards, invitations, ads, informational booklets, press packages and press releases. This highly informative and practical workshop breaks through the obstacles practitioners face when preparing these materials. It begins with a guided meditation that helps participants move into a relaxed state. By maintaining this state of calmness, participants are able to channel their innate wisdom into effective marketing presentations.

IGNITE THE SPARK OF CREATIVITY
A four-hour workshop on
Presentation Skills

There is a sacred place within each one of us where true creativity springs forth. The process through which we can move into that space and maintain access whenever we want is a muscle which can be developed. Through improvisational theater techniques, practitioners will learn how to tap into that wellspring, ignite the spark of creativity, and then act and react from a place of strength and confidence.

Current, real-ife situations will be reenacted by participants, so they begin to look objectively at the way they present themselves in everyday situations. The enactments are reviewed by other participants and options are openly discussed.

The workshop becomes a catalyst for letting go of unnecessary habits, guards, and inhibitions as we explore new and interesting ways to present ourselves.

Initially, the exercises will seem easy. However, as the day progresses, the exercises become more challenging and complex. The result of this concentrated effort is that participants become more agile and flexible.

Using improvisational games, the imagination gets stimulated, the intuition gets strengthened. The exercises become a powerful tool for growth, so that participants begin to trust instinctively that the choices they make are the right ones — for every situation.

For prices and availability, e-mail andreapr@aol.com

KEYNOTE SPEAKING

Andrea is a dynamic, entertaining presenter. Her strong theatrical background adds to her versatile speaking style. Her enthusiasm and love shine through as she speaks passionately and sincerely to the challenges practitioners and healing centers face.

Each speech can be modified to run from a half hour long to two and a half hours, depending on your needs.

CONSULTATIONS

Andrea offers a two- to four-hour consultation for individual practitioners, healing centers and professional associations.

This one-on-one session, whether on the phone or in person, is an intimate process through which Andrea looks closely at all past and present outreach efforts — marketing materials, events, media exposure, articles to date.

Andrea assesses all efforts and provides each client with a clear understanding of their audience — who their audience is, or needs to be — and how to reach them. She provides a practical strategy so that clients are able to move through obstacles, gracefully, and into the vision of their future.

Although her approach is eminently practical, she reframes the approach conceptually, out-of-the-box, bringing her clients delightful new approaches to old ways of thinking. Through the creation of new paradigms, she aids practitioners and centers by enabling them to transform their own understanding of what they have to offer.

To schedule a consultation or speech, e-mail andreapr@aol.com

ABOUT THE AUTHOR

Andrea Adler's love and respect for this distinctive audience, coupled with her extensive PR and marketing background, makes her the ideal facilitator to reveal the strategies that have been the basis for her successful career.

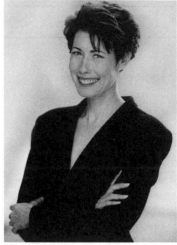

Andrea has been a marketing and public-relations consultant for over 20 years, promoting and marketing holistic practitioners, healing centers, Internet companies, multimedia and artistic ventures (fashion, music, theatrical) throughout the U.S.

As an author, she has written *PR for the Holistic Healer: A Handbook on Promoting and Marketing Your Practice,* and *Creating an Abundant Practice: A Spiritual and Practical Guide for Holistic Practitioners and Healing Centers,* as well as articles for *Body Mind Spirit* magazine, *The Times Herald Record,* and *Uno Mismo*, a New Age magazine in Buenos Aires. Ms. Adler wrote Herbal Life's first audio promotional tape, and marketing collateral for Bread for the World, EDF (Environmental Defense Fund), City Harvest, Food for Thought and Co-op America.

Andrea presents workshops and keynote addresses at healing centers, schools, businesses, professional organizations and top corporations throughout America. She is currently based in Santa Fe, New Mexico.